5·1·79

Life Begins at Forty

How to make sure you enjoy middle age

Life Begins at Forty

How to make sure you enjoy middle age

Ann Burkitt

Illustrated by Val Biro

Hutchinson Benham, London
In association with the Health Education Council

Hutchinson Benham Ltd
3 Fitzroy Square, London W1

An imprint of the Hutchinson Group

London Melbourne Sydney Auckland
Wellington Johannesburg and agencies
throughout the world

Text © The Health Education Council 1977
Illustrations © Hutchinson Benham Ltd 1977
First published 1977

Set in Monotype Times
Printed in Great Britain by litho at
The Anchor Press Ltd, and bound by
Wm Brendon & Son Ltd, both of
Tiptree, Essex

ISBN 0 09 129101 1

Contents

2048834

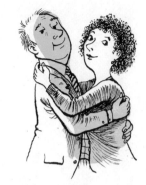

Life Begins
at Forty

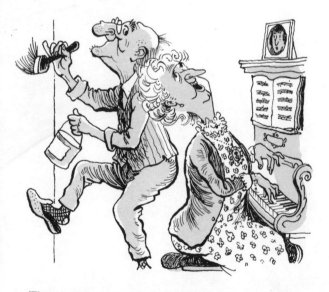

'There are men and women of eighty ready to tackle any new task'

Introduction

How old you feel is really very much a state of mind and outlook. When you are sixteen, middle age starts at thirty, and when you are thirty middle age is still a long way off. There are people who as teenagers have set ideas, often thought to be a sign of growing old. On the other hand there are men and women of eighty ready to tackle any new task or to look in a fresh way at any problem to be solved. When everything is going well most people feel younger than they are, but when things are difficult and they don't know how to cope with their problems it is likely that they feel older.

Society judges the same age in many different ways as well. A man of forty-five can be a middle-aged father, a young grandfather, an elderly footballer, or an extremely young Prime Minister.

How people think they should act at different ages and in a variety of situations is determined to a large extent by how their society thinks they should act. In some countries, particularly in rural areas, when a girl marries she puts on dark colours and is supposed to act in a mature and sober way. In Britain, and even more in the USA, women of sixty or more wear the latest fashions and make-up.

Most of us have set ideas about other people and how they should behave. And in the same way there are many set ideas about middle age. People are told that all women going through the menopause are difficult, have hot flushes, and will never enjoy sex again; that men at forty start to look for younger women; that sex after fifty is not nice; that it is not safe to give jobs needing adaptability to men over forty-five. When these statements are examined closely it can be seen how untrue they are for most individuals and that they reflect the opinion and character of the speaker rather than reality.

Middle age is most often thought of as the years between forty and sixty. It is the time when many people are learning to be parents of adolescents, grandparents for the first time, and nursemaids to elderly sick parents. For some people it may mean the satisfaction of getting to the top of the ladder, for others the realization that they are never going to get any further; for some it may even mean redundancy, and for all it is a preparation for retirement. That is if you look at it as a tailing off, but for many people middle age is just the beginning. It may be the start of a new career or back to the books and the student life. It may be the long-awaited chance to take up again hobbies and interests which had to be given up while a family was being raised. It may be the first chance to travel.

For many people middle age is the high plateau of their life. They have learnt to come to terms with themselves, they know their possibilities and they have faced up to their weaknesses. This is the period in which most working men and women can be of most value. Their experience, knowledge and maturity can be of great sevice to society in whatever job or position they may be. It's not for nothing that many middle-aged people would describe themselves as being in the prime of life.

We hope this book will help to dispel some of the myths and fears about middle age and the menopause and help you to enjoy what can and should be a very happy and rewarding time of life.

1. Marriage and family relationships

Statistics show that most people who marry, marry between the ages of twenty and thirty, and they will have completed the size of the family they want during the first five to ten years of marriage. With younger and younger marriages becoming general, especially for girls, and with more people reaching old age, marriage has become a long-term contract in the way it never was before. How many Victorian couples celebrated their golden wedding anniversary?

These tendencies have had far-reaching consequences on marriage, on family relationships, and on the role of women in society. The working woman has always been with us. What is new is that she is now better educated, may be working outside the home, and is demanding equal rights with men.

Understanding children

Children growing up, leaving home, getting married and having their own children produce new situations to which their parents must adjust. Frequently a mother reaches the menopause just when her children are going through their own hormonal changes during adolescence, and this can make for a very stormy time. If people at least understand that there is an underlying biological basis for their behaviour it may help them to be more tolerant of one another.

There have been many books written examining the relationship between the teenager and his or her parents. Having attractive teenage children who are only just coming to terms with their own sexuality creates not only the usual arguments of how much freedom and control you should impose, but also the realization that you are growing older yourself.

Parents who tease a son or daughter about their hair style, friends or political ideas should stop and ask themselves 'Do they really need taking down a peg or is it because I resent the chances they have which were denied to me?'

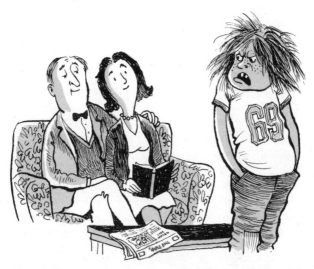

Adolescence is known to be a time for trying out new ideas and scoffing at the old, but parents can take heart in the fact that a survey among secondary school children showed that over 90 per cent of them considered their home and parents to be the most important thing in their lives. Once they become independent and start to live their own adult lives, most children realize even more clearly the value of their parents.

Caring for parents

Middle-aged people, and not just those who are married, usually also have a responsibility to their own parents. Before industrialization and the move to live huddled in large towns, families were larger, generations merged into one another and there were always unmarried daughters, cousins or some poorer relations around who helped in the house, helped with the children and helped with those grandparents who survived into old age.

Most of us now live in small family units, and houses are rarely designed to provide space for grandparents. Even so, we are not a nation that shuts our old people away in homes, judging by a recent survey which showed that the majority of elderly parents either live close to or with one of their children. But while we realize the need for showing love and affection to young people, this is often forgotten when it comes to the old.

When children marry or leave home and establish their own life, the parents have to re-learn the art of living their own independent lives. If because of death, illness or lack of finance the independent families are reunited, there must be a great readjustment on both sides. The mother may find it very difficult to accept her daughter or daughter-in-law's role as a principal housekeeper; she may disapprove of her ideas of child-rearing. The early period of settling needs special tolerance on both sides. Loss of a lifelong partner can completely bewilder the one who is left, usually the wife, and make her difficult to live with.

Many elderly people have disabilities and it is worth knowing that help such as a district nurse and special aid from the local authority is available. Elderly people may qualify to register as disabled persons. GPs or the local Social Services Department will explain about the various kinds of grant available.

Grandparents and their grandchildren can often achieve a special relationship. They both have so much to give each other in love and understanding. If grandparents are accused of spoiling, it may be because they are allowed to show their love or concern only in material ways. Of course grandparents occasionally feel resentful if they are constantly used as unpaid baby-sitters. But with a bit of tactful organization the parents could enable the grandparents to share the children, with mutual benefits.

Single people

There is another relationship which must be considered – that of the parent and the single child. We are using the word single here to mean not just those who have never married, but those who have been deserted, separated, divorced or widowed and who are now alone.

Many people choose not to marry, or never have the opportunity, or forgo marriage because of family demands. Except for the age group now under twenty years, there have always been more women than men available for marriage, and with men having a higher death rate and shorter life expectancy than women, a widow or divorcee has less chance of re-marriage than a man.

Then there is that group of men and women in our society who are homosexual. Many do not realize that they are, have no sexual experience and never feel the need to marry. Some, particularly men, because of social disapproval and the laws of our society, may live only with others like themselves and have lost all contact with their families. Others may have fairly successful marriages at the same time. Yet others will form permanent homosexual relationships, having most of the characteristics of a marriage between a man and a woman except children.

Single people, particularly women, may have a special problem in coping with elderly parents. Married brothers and sisters immersed in their own children's needs frequently leave their unmarried sister to cope alone. This may impose a heavy financial strain on the daughter, particularly as women's jobs are notoriously badly paid in comparison with men's (in spite of the Equal Pay Act), and she may find it difficult to gain promotion if she is also coping with sick parents at home. This is an important social problem. The Society for the Single Woman and Her Dependants estimates that there are a quarter of a million women coping with elderly parents, and is campaigning for more financial help for them. When, because of

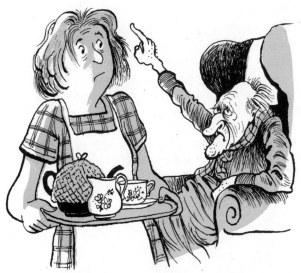

'Single people, particularly women, may have a special problem in coping with elderly parents'

the death of the parent, the children have to reconstruct a new life for themselves, they may find it very difficult.

Fortunately there are now opportunities for middle-aged people to start new careers such as social work and nursing. There are some colleges that cater especially for mature students, and the Open University should provide a spur to many people to start their education afresh. Those who keep their minds keen and alert are likely to be better able to cope with their later independence both emotionally and intellectually than did their parents, who suffered from restricted financial and intellectual outlets.

Drifting apart

If you marry at twenty, at forty-five you will be having your silver wedding anniversary and still have maybe another thirty years of married life ahead of you. Fifty years is a long time for two people to live togther in perfect harmony, and not surprisingly an increasing number of marriages do break up. sometimes for what seem to be trivial reasons.

During the course of time some couples become so used to one another that they hardly notice their partner's existence until something unusual happens and they realize their plight. Then one or other may seek a way out to escape the sheer boredom.

Small cracks in a relationship are easy to gloss over. It is easy to find excuses in the demands of children and a taxing job for why so little time is spent together. And falling alseep in front of the television every night ensures little conversation.

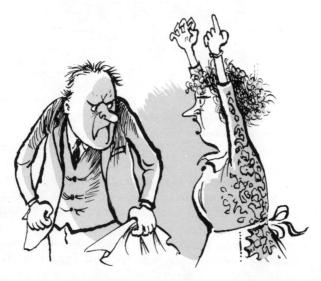

Stress in a relationship may build up very gradually until resentment breaks out in the form of constant nagging and rows. The wife may find everything too much trouble and neglect the household chores; the fact that she also works outside the home may not persuade the husband that he should do some housework and he spends all his time away from home, so creating a recipe for disaster.

Many marriages are ruined by jealousy. But if a couple have a solid, honest relationship where there is mutual respect and trust and they can discuss things together, then even if one or other of them does find another person attractive and interesting, their relationship is hardly likely to break up. They both know they have too much to lose.

It is clear that many people, especially young people, enter marriage with unreal expectations of what married life will be like. They have little idea of managing money and the hard realities of running a home, and may see marriage as an escape from an unhappy home or a dull job. When it turns out to be not the bed of roses they expected they are at a complete loss. The many letters to the agony columns of women's and teenage magazines show how often this happens.

Situations like this are all too common, but it is often difficult to know what to do about them. Each marriage is a unique relationship and no one can provide a set of rules which will ensure instant success. Some manage to survive in spite of the rows and problems; others break up. Individual counselling has provided help for many marriages and the work of the Marriage Guidance Council is well known. What is not realized is that the probation service will also provide a counselling service and advice on financial rights.

Divorce is the final resort of an unhappy marriage, and the latest divorce laws permit the ending of a marriage so long as there is evidence that it has irretrievably broken down. The use of the word irretrievably does suggest that the state has some duty to help prevent couples ending in the divorce courts, and financial grants are made towards the work of the Marriage Guidance Council. Where a divorce or a separation seems the only possible outcome, the Citizens' Advice Bureau will supply a list of local solicitors on request.

On the positive side, marriage has never been more popular. There is a higher percentage of the population married than at any other time since records have been kept, and those who do get divorced often make a successful second marriage.

2. The menopause

The whole period during which a woman's body is changing from a state of possible fertility to infertility is properly called the 'climacteric' – usually known as 'the change of life'. The ceasing of the menstrual periods is called 'the menopause'. But because 'the change of life' sounds so alarming and final (the phrase must surely have been invented by a male doctor with a grudge against women) we shall call this whole period 'the menopause'. It usually occurs from approximately forty-five to fifty-five, but may start as early as thirty-five and end as late as fifty-eight.

Growth and development is not something which stops at eighteen, but it is a continuing process throughout our lives. The ending of a woman's periods, like their beginning, is one of the milestones of the body's gradual change.

Just as it is impossible to know when a girl's periods will start, it is impossible to know when they will end. The menopause may start at forty or not until the mid-fifties. For some women periods may stop abruptly; for others they will be irregular and then gradually tail off. The irregularity of the periods may lead a woman to fear an unwanted pregnancy but this is unlikely providing she is taking proper precautions (birth control is fully discussed in a later chapter).

The menopause is a subject which is widely talked and joked about. It is the period of life which many women dread because of exaggerated tales of what happens to friends and relatives, and because of the general belief that once a woman ceases to menstruate she is no longer a real woman.

In biological terms the menopause means a woman can no longer have a baby, but it does not mean the end of her sexual life. To understand what actually happens in a woman's body

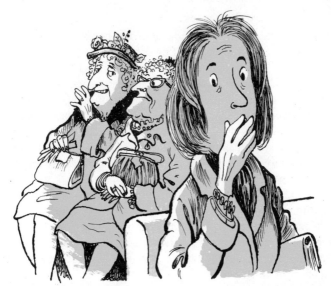

'The menopause is a subject which is widely talked and joked about'

to cause all these changes, we must first look at how her reproductive system works.

How a woman's reproductive system works

A woman's reproductive system (see also diagram on page 64) consists of two ovaries which from her birth contain the cells of all the eggs she will ever produce, two fallopian tubes leading from the ovaries to the uterus (or womb), and the vagina which leads from her uterus to the outside of her body. On the outside are the labia – the soft folds of skin which protect the opening of the vagina – and the opening of the urethra, the tube down which the urine passes. At the join of the labia is a small pea-shaped lump called the clitoris, the main centre of sexual pleasure for women.

From the time of birth the ovaries produce two female hormones called oestrogen and progesterone. At puberty more of these hormones are produced to bring about the body changes such as the enlargement of the breasts and the hips and the start of the periods. For the first time the eggs in the ovaries start to ripen, and at roughly twenty-eight-day intervals an egg is released into one of the fallopian tubes. At the same time the spongy wall of the uterus has become rich with blood in case the egg is fertilized and should need nourishment. If fertilization does not take place the tiny egg dies, and the unrequired spongy lining is discharged from the body. This is a woman's monthly period. Not everybody's periods are regular; some may be very irregular, and unfamiliar events such as a new job, or moving house, can temporarily upset the body rhythm.

When a woman becomes pregnant the balance of the female hormones changes. No eggs are released nor do periods occur during pregnancy, although occasionally a slight period may occur in the early months.

What happens during the menopause?

During the menopause the balance of the two female hormones is once more readjusted. In some people this happens easily. In others the balance is sometimes thrown out of gear, and it's this that causes the side effects which so many women fear. Some women in fact have no trouble at all.

There are a variety of ways in which periods finish:

1. In some women they stop suddenly – one month you have a period, the next month nothing.

2. More usually periods become small and gradually tail off.

3. The time between periods becomes longer and longer or the periods become irregular and tail off.

This tailing-off process may take several years.

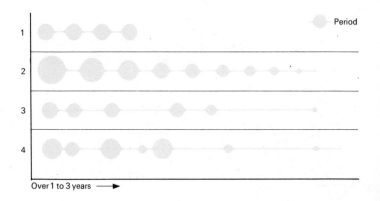

Four ways in which periods can stop

Side effects of the menopause

Hot flushes

These may start several years before there is any alteration in the frequency of the periods and they affect different women in different ways. In one they may feel like a wave of heat sweeping up through the body and leaving her sweating. She may be woken at night and need to push off the bedclothes. In another woman the sensation may be slight. Hot flushes in the day may be brought on by annoyance or confusion. The flushes are caused by blood rushing to the surface blood vessels in the skin. The blood supply is controlled by the sympathetic nervous system which cannot be consciously controlled. During the menopause this system may become for a time upset. causing the blood vessels to expand suddenly (flushing) and then causing them to close down, cutting the supply to the

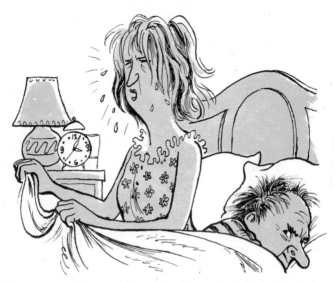

'She may be woken at night and need to push off the bedclothes'

surface vessels. This is the reason for paleness and cold hands and feet when the rest of the body is warm.

Skin

The skin may become drier than usual and, in particular, an irritation may start on the skin between the legs, and normal secretion of the vagina dry up. (This is discussed later in the book.)

Nervous symptoms

Many women during the menopause complain of tiredness, and an inability to concentrate on a job. Others may feel anxiety, numbness and irritability. Occasionally, and particularly at night, some women may feel as if the heart is beating unevenly (palpitations). There are now treatments which the doctor can prescribe to lessen these symptoms.

Headaches

Headaches are not uncommon. Many people overlook the fact that their eyesight changes with age, and that their headaches may be due to either a need for glasses, or a change of the ones which they are wearing. It is important to tell the optician about any drugs being taken, as some drugs do affect the eyesight. For example, the pill may make it difficult to wear contact lenses.

Migraine can start at any stage of life but can occur for the first time during the menopause. Migraine headaches are often accompanied by visual disturbances, nausea and even vomiting. It is now thought that there could be a connection between diet and migraine and it might help migraine sufferers to think what they ate just before they had their last attack, in order to see if there is any connection between certain types of food and the onset of a migraine. Persistent migraine sufferers can get help from the Migraine Trust (see end of book for the address), as well as from their GP.

Digestion

Some women develop flatulence, constipation, and a swollen tummy (abdominal distension), but these are probably due more to lack of exercise and a sensible diet than the menopause. If the symptoms persist, the doctor should be consulted.

Obesity

Obesity in middle age is a problem of both men and women and it is not confined to the menopause. Occasionally, it may be due to hormonal imbalance, but it is far more likely to be due to eating the wrong sort of food or too much of it.

Softening of the bones

After the menopause women start to lose calcium (the hardening material) from their bones. It is more rapid in some women than others but it is a long-term process. This is why elderly women are prone to broken bones, especially wrists and the neck of the long upper bone of the leg.

Mood changes

All of us, male and female, at all stages of our lives, experience changes of mood. If others think well of us, if we have just done a job well, or we know that we look good, we tend to be in a good mood. If things are not going well it is difficult to feel happy.

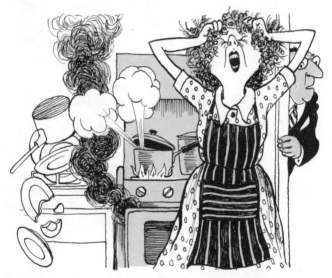

'If things are not going well it is difficult to feel happy'

Some women describe a sensation of feeling like cotton wool, a sense of losing control of their emotions and feelings and because of this have an increased fear of mental illness at this time. Most women do experience swings of mood partly because of hormonal changes and also because the menopause often coincides with other family upheavals and changes.

Children leaving home, elderly parents needing help or falling ill, or the reorganization of a working life may all contribute to a feeling of depression. Whether or not the depression continues depends on the woman's ability with the help of her family and friends to adjust to the new situation, and most people do adjust very well. Some may find they need medical help for a short time to overcome the feeling of depression, and then they are back again to their readjusted lives.

The important thing to remember is that the menopause is a normal part of body development and that a great many problems are blamed on it which are coincidental. Of course women do have very real problems due to the menopause and it is always a good idea to talk these over with another person, especially another sympathetic woman, or if you think you need medical treatment go to the family doctor. In the back of this book you will find a list of addresses of organizations which can help with various problems.

Hormonal replacement therapy

Hormonal Replacement Therapy (HRT) is widely used in the USA and increasingly used in Britain. It has been hailed as a biological revolution for women. There are many who are convinced that it is the solution to the menopause and others who feel there may be dangers, so that caution should be used.

Basically it means replacing the natural oestrogen, no longer being made in large quantities by the woman's body, with oestrogen by tablet. There is no doubt that HRT considerably reduces side effects of the menopause. Women on HRT feel better, their skin and hair improves, the normal secretions of the vagina return and hot flushes lessen.

With such results, no wonder thousands of women are enthusiastic; so why are not all women on the menopause put automatically on to HRT? First of all, many women's bodies go on making enough oestrogen, so that they have few or no side effects of the menopause except for the loss of periods.

Secondly, some doctors say that HRT has not been in long enough use for possible side effects to show and they point out that the oestrogen widely used is not natural oestrogen which is a lot more expensive. Some people question the cost of HRT to the National Health Service, although this seems a pointless argument when you consider the millions of pounds spent on tranquillizers, skin creams and sleeping pills to cope with the side effects which use of HRT would solve.

There are now special Menopause Clinics being set up in different parts of the country which are carrying out research into the use of HRT. Their addresses are in the back of the book. Ask your doctor what he or she thinks.

You may find you have a local Well Woman Clinic that is also interested in HRT. The more people ask about it, the more interest will be taken in it by the medical profession.

If you would like to know more about this subject, *No Change* by Wendy Cooper, published by Hutchinson, is a comprehensive, enthusiastic summary of the treatment.

What to do about the menopause

1. All women do have a menopause, so accept that it is a normal stage of every female's development. It is not the end of being a woman or being sexy; it is the beginning of a new phase in your life.

2. Having said that, if you do have side effects don't let people tell you it's all in the mind. It is not.

3. Talk to your partner and family. Explain how you feel and why, so that they can be understanding.

4. If the side effects are distressing go to your GP. If he or she is not helpful, ask if you can be referred to a Menopause Clinic or ask your local Family Planning Clinic if they have a doctor who specializes in this area.

5. Treatment of and interest in the menopause is very new, so you can't expect all doctors to be interested and knowledge-able. If you feel the service for menopausal women in your

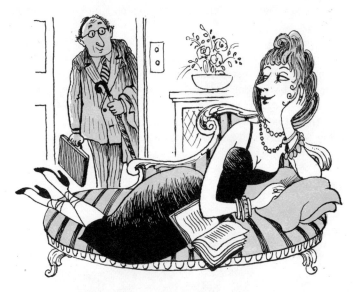

'It is not the end of being a woman or being sexy'

area is inadequate, write to your community health council. They are there to look after your interests. Ask them to look into the matter. Their address will be in your telephone book, or you can ask Directory Inquiries.

6. In the list of addresses in the back you may find an organization which caters for your own particular need. Your own health district may run Well Women or Menopause Clinics who could give special help. Telephone their main office for information.

Do men have a menopause?

Although boys go through obvious body changes during adolescence, men do not have a menopause in the same way as women. Some researchers have suggested that there may be minor changes apart from the gradual ageing process, although men do not have hot flushes and obvious signs of a physical change.

No one has investigated the middle-aged man in the same way as they have the middle-aged woman. We know that men go on producing sperm because of the numbers of quite elderly men who have become fathers, but with increasing age the numbers of sperm produced grow less. Apart from this there is nothing that compares with the ending of a woman's periods. (They do have a gradual decrease of the male hormone testosterone.)

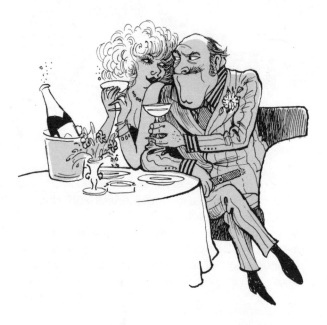

There is a popular picture of the middle-aged man as being ready for his last fling, getting itchy feet and having an upsurge of sexual desire. There would appear to be no physical reason for this and it is more likely the result of the influence of Hollywood and wishful thinking.

In a small piece of research on the attitudes towards middle age of men over forty years old several interesting points emerged. Although the men had clear ideas about middle age they did not want to admit that they had reached the state, and felt uncomfortable with the idea. Often they would only admit its reality to themselves after a dramatic experience such as being told by their foreman that they were being put on a different job because they could no longer cope with the one they had, or because they were passed over for promotion and their age given as a reason.

Although many of the men admitted to being unfit, keeping fit was considered sissy. They were frightened by the idea of being ill and helpless and yet did not want to alter their diet, especially the number of pints of beer or their smoking habits.

Three sorts of things were feared – being downgraded or losing a job, impotence and dependence, retirement and death. Many of the men were fatalistic, feeling that there was nothing they could do to alter their lives.

Fears about jobs

Many different types of skilled work demand regular medical check-ups. Men feared failing these tests and being forced to take jobs of lower grades. Men in demanding administrative or management positions were well aware of the bright young men waiting to step into their shoes. All the men knew others who had once held 'a real man's job' and who were now in a low grade position.

Impotence and dependence

While a gradual decline in sexual potency was accepted as inevitable there was a general fear of loss of power and author-ity in the family, particularly situations such as 'becoming dependent on my children' and 'turning into a vegetable for my wife to look after'. There was a particular fear of these things happening as the result of an accident or a stroke.

Retirement

Few men consciously prepare for retirement. Work is considered to be the meaning of life and yet many find their work boring and repetitive, providing little mental stimulation.

At a time of rapid technological change, when re-training, redundancy and unemployment are possibilities in many people's lives, whether on the shop floor, in management or the professions, the need for someone to care about you as a person has never been greater.

There is little doubt that the husband's attitude to his wife during her menopause is of great importance. It may not always be easy for him to understand her moods and tension and her possible temporary lack of interest in love-making. But from the results of the survey shown above it is clear that men have their problems too. And just as a woman needs her husband's understanding, so he needs hers. If his wife is concerned and sympathetic the man is more likely to adapt to the changes in his situation and accept the need to care for his health too.

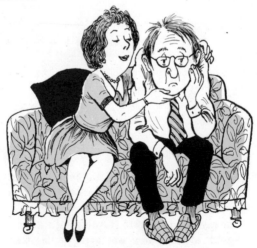

'It is clear that men have their problems too'

3. The sexual relationship

Sexual intercourse is a natural human activity. In some societies young girls and men are taught sexual techniques by their elders, and although they may not know a great deal about anatomy and physiology, the delights of love for them are not a terrifying mystery as they are to many people in our own society.

Reaching the menopause is not a reason for the end of a satisfying sexual life unless a woman believes wholeheartedly that intercourse is only for producing children. Very few people really do believe this. In fact the period of life after the menopause can be the most sexually satisfying of all, secure from the worries of pregnancy and the demands of small children.

Sexual feelings are very much a state of mind and do not depend on age. What is important is the relationship between the couple. Those who have a spontaneous, easy relationship and who are able to talk about their feelings to one another should be able to cope with the adjustments to new situations. Those couples who never discuss anything which is really important to them, especially their sexual life, can take the easy way out and use an operation such as sterilization, the menopause or the children leaving home as the scapegoat for why their marriage isn't working or their sex life gives no satisfaction.

Very few middle-aged people today have had the advantage of a good, constructive sex education. Although we may know a great deal about many other subjects, very few of us have been educated about ourselves. So it is not surprising that there are many myths and fears about our bodies, babies and sex, and particularly about what is abnormal.

There are many people whose lives have been difficult, miserable and lonely because they thought there was something wrong with them. The Kinsey Report did a great service to Anglo-American society by showing that many of the so-called abnormal practices such as masturbation were practised by such a large number of people that they were in fact perfectly normal.

Our society has encouraged the belief that sexual intercourse must allow the man to reach his climax inside the woman's vagina. In fact at times the law has tried to prevent other forms of intercourse such as sodomy where the back passage is used. (Before good birth control became available this was often used to prevent pregnancy.) Goodness only knows how the authorities thought they could enforce the law.

Yet there are many ways in which a man and woman can give pleasure and comfort to one another. There are times when it is uncomfortable or even impossible to have full intercourse, such as at certain times during pregnancy, or straight after having a baby or an operation. There is no reason why a man and a woman should not still give each other comfort, love and sexual pleasure by other means, such as mutual masturbation. There can be no perversions in love-making when two people care and are concerned about each other.

Sometimes illness may make a couple take a fresh look at their sexual lives. There are some medical conditions where individual couples may need specific help, such as after a coronary thrombosis. If the husband has been ill this may be the first time the woman has thought to adopt an active role as in the woman above the man position. This can give pleasure to both with little physical strain on the man.

Until some studies were done by two American scientists called Masters and Johnson, no one had really scientifically examined sexual intercourse. Their results showed that the clitoris was the main source of a female climax, not the vagina as people had always believed. If men knew and paid more attention to this fact there would be greater mutual satisfaction.

The reduction in the female hormone oestrogen during and after the menopause may cause the natural secretions of the vagina to dry up, making sexual intercourse difficult. This can be helped by hormone replacement therapy (described elsewhere) and by using KY lubricating jelly, available from chemists.

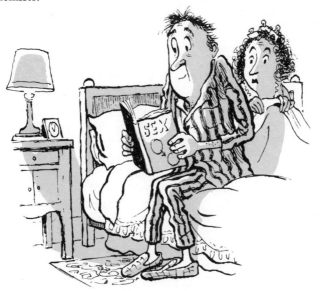

'There are many books available on sexual techniques'

There are many books available on sexual techniques, some excellent and some not very helpful. A list of the most useful ones is given at the back of this book. Books can be very helpful as guide-lines, but the real secret is the loving, giving relationship. Sexual ability and enjoyment depend on the couple concerned rather than on their age. If a couple does have sexual problems which can't be sorted out just by talking together, the Family Planning Association and the Marriage Guidance Council run special marital problems sessions and they will be only too glad to help in such cases.

Single people have varying sexual needs just as married people do. They might find that masturbation is a satisfactory outlet; they may have affairs, often of many years' length, and most have built up a satisfactory life with a job, friends and family. Not everybody has a well-developed maternal sense and they may find being an aunt or uncle without the problems of parenthood enjoyable.

Love-making

How often two people make love is an individual matter, but that it is one which causes concern is indicated by the number of letters printed in women's magazines asking for advice. Men and women do have different amounts of sexual desire. Research has shown that women show marked fluctuations in their needs, closely following their hormonal pattern. In the first years of marriage love-making will probably be more frequent than later on, no matter at what age the couple marry. Some couples will make love once a night, every night of the week. Others will make love twice on a Saturday because they can sleep in on Sunday. It may depend on the husband's and wife's jobs. Shift work will affect how often and when a couple make love. Modern life with long journeys to work, TV, the needs of children, a hundred and one things will also affect the frequency of intercourse. It is a good idea sometimes for a couple to take a look at all their activities. Making time just to sit down and have a talk about things can often solve a lot of problems.

Pregnancy in middle age

A few women enter middle age looking forward to having a planned and longed for first baby, and others to whom the thought of having another baby before it is too late seems very attractive. There is no medical reason why a woman of over forty should not have a baby if she is fit and well and if she wants one, although there are certain factors she should consider and discuss with her doctor before embarking on pregnancy. As long as she makes sure she sees her doctor and midwife regularly, pregnancy should be as enjoyable as if she were twenty-five.

But there are many middle-aged women who dread the thought of another baby and who become worried and depressed when their periods become irregular in case it means pregnancy. The menopausal woman needs the best possible birth-control advice. There are many women who find themselves faced with an unwanted pregnancy – and not just married women. In 1971, 1164 illegitimate babies, live and still births were born to women in England and Wales between the ages of forty and forty-nine. Of course, not all illegitimate babies are unwanted. Many of these babies were probably born to couples living in a stable relationship but not legally married, or to women who were financially secure and wanted a baby. But in that group of women there may have been many who were desperately worried and without any idea of where to go for help. The sixteen-year-old pregnant girl usually creates sympathy, but it is so easy for society to dismiss the older woman with a shrug and 'she should have known better'. Imagine how difficult it must be for the divorced woman with two almost grown-up children discovering to her horror that because of one careless night she is pregnant.

2048834

Where to get help

Whether you are married or single the first thing you should do if you suspect an unwanted pregnancy is to consult your GP. If the pregnancy is confirmed he will refer you to a consultant if you feel an abortion would be the best solution. If your GP is not helpful you have a right to ask for a second opinion. If you have any difficulties there are addresses at the back of the book of people who can help you in the decision as to whether you should have an abortion or keep the child.

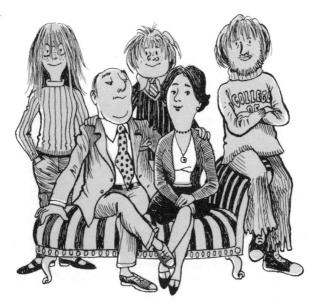

'It is likely that they will have all the children they want'

Contraception

Conception is the fertilization of the woman's egg by the man's sperm. Contraception simply means preventing this from happening. Most couples nowadays use some form of contraception to make sure they have a baby only when they want it, and don't have more children than they can look after.

For middle-aged couples the use of a really effective method of birth control is particularly important, since it is likely they will have all the children they want and a further pregnancy would be particularly unwelcome.

Any method of contraception can be used, but because of the menopause there are special points to consider. It is impossible to say exactly when a woman becomes completely infertile after her periods stop. Research has shown that even after the finish of periods an egg may occasionally ripen and be released into the fallopian tubes as it would be during the normal monthly cycle. This is because the two female hormones which control the release of the egg have not yet completely readjusted themselves to their new balance.

Doctors advise women under fifty that to be completely free of worry about pregnancy during the menopause a reliable form of contraception should be continuously used for at least two years after the last period. For women over fifty a year is sufficient. These precautions will ensure that there will be no worries about possible pregnancy.

When most of today's middle-aged couples married, the only forms of contraception available were the sheath, some-times called a French letter, rubber or condom (for the man), the Dutch cap, foaming tablets and creams (for the woman). Sheaths, creams, aerosol foams and tablets are still easily obtainable from the chemist and surgical supply shops. They need no medical supervision and have no side effects. If the couple have used these methods successfully and are happy with them, then these are perfectly satisfactory methods for the menopause so long as they are used every time the couple make love.

Methods of birth control

Chemical creams, foams or jellies

These are put into the woman's vagina to stop or kill the sperms before they can meet the egg cell. There are several kinds of chemicals.

Aerosol foam is the most effective of all chemical barriers when it is used on its own. It is packed under pressure in a small container and expelled into the vagina by a plunger, filled from the container.

Jellies or creams are squeezed on to the cap before it is put in the sex passage, or are pushed direct into the vagina by means of a special applicator.

Soluble tablets or pessaries have to be put as far up the vagina as possible just before the sex act.

None of these birth-control chemicals is completely reliable by itself, so most people only use them with a cap or French letter.

The condom (sheath)

Condoms, sheaths or French letters are the most widely used method of birth control. They can be bought from most chemists, surgical stores and barbers, but to be sure of the best quality look out for the BS kite mark on the packet.

Condoms should be rolled on to the erect penis before any contact with the woman takes place. To be doubly sure the woman should also put a chemical barrier into her vagina just in case the French letter should leak or burst.

After the love-making the man must withdraw his penis while it is still erect so that the condom does not slip off. A new condom should be used each time the sex act takes place – unless the thicker kind, which can be washed and used again, is used. There are no side effects with the sheath. In fact many men prefer it because they like to feel they are in control of their partner's fertility.

The cap (diaphragm)

Caps have been popular for many years. They are completely harmless and very reliable if used correctly.

The woman places the cap, which is made of soft rubber, in her vagina so that it covers the mouth of the womb and prevents the sperms from meeting the egg cell. She should always smear some birth-control cream or jelly on both sides of the cap to prevent any sperms from getting round the rim and into the neck of her womb.

There are many shapes and sizes of cap, so a doctor must choose the right size for each woman. Once she has been fitted she will be shown how to put it in and take it out. The cap should be put in before intercourse and taken out at any convenient time six hours or more afterwards.

The pill (oral contraceptive)

The pill works by preventing the woman's body from releasing an egg cell each month. If there is no egg cell she cannot become pregnant.

The pill has to be taken on a regular monthly cycle, and the doctor will explain exactly how to take it. If instructions are followed completely the pill is virtually 100 per cent reliable. The pill is only provided on a doctor's prescription. You can go either to your own GP or to a Family Planning Clinic.

Some women may get a headache, or sick feeling, or weight increase when they first go on the pill, but these and any other

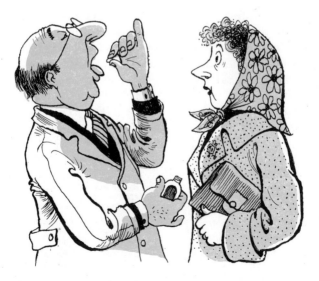

'The doctor will explain exactly how to take it'

troubles should clear up in a little while. A very few women cannot use the pill at all.

Women who take the pill stand a slightly higher risk of developing blood clots than those who are not on the pill. But the risk is still very small compared with the risks attached to pregnancy which themselves are small due to medical supervision. Millions of women throughout the world are now taking the pill because it is the most effective and convenient method of birth control available.

Although the pill has many advantages, especially that of providing peace of mind, it has one problem for the woman approaching the menopause. How does she know when she has got there? Because the pill takes over control of her periods a woman can go right through the menopause and not know it. Of course this could be seen as an advantage, but most doctors like to take a woman of forty-five and over off the pill for a few months to see if her periods have stopped. During this time she will be given another form of contraceptive to use, and if she still has her periods she can go back on the pill again.

The pill has been a thoroughly researched form of contraception, but doctors freely admit we still don't know everything about it. All women on the pill whatever their age, but especially over forty, should make sure they have a regular six-monthly check of their weight, blood pressure and breasts and a yearly cyto test. If your GP doesn't do it, then ask why not. If he or she still doesn't provide this service then go to a Family Planning Clinic that does.

The loop (IUD or coil)

The loop is a tiny shape of soft plastic or soft plastic-covered fine copper wire which is fitted into the woman's womb by a specially trained doctor. There is no need for an anaesthetic and the whole thing only takes a couple of minutes. Once the loop is in there is no need to worry about it except for checking that it is still there after a period. The loop is put completely inside the uterus, but a very fine thread is left hanging through the uterus opening, the cervix and the vagina. This can be felt by a finger but in no way interferes with love-making. As long as the loop is in place it will nearly always prevent pregnancy.

For about three months after the loop has been inserted the periods are usually heavier, but then they settle down. The advantage for the menopausal woman is that she knows exactly where she is, which is not the case with the pill. The loop is a good method of birth control particularly for the middle-aged woman, but it is not suitable for everybody. The doctor will need to examine the woman internally before he or she will recommend the loop. This method has a high success rate for the woman who finds it suitable.

The rhythm method (safe period)

The rhythm method or safe period is used by a great many people and not always for religious reasons. Biologically there

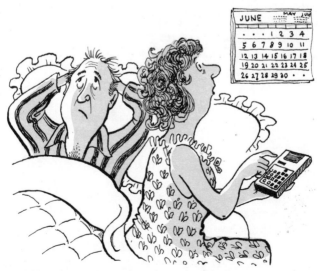

'It would be better to forget the safe period altogether'

are only about four days in the monthly cycle when it is possible to conceive. So long as love-making does not take place on those days there is no need to use any form of contraception. This would be fine as long as periods were absolutely regular so that the calculation of these days was easy, and also if Nature (which likes to make sure of reproductive success) had not ensured that a woman has monthly peaks of sexual desire, one of them during the fertile days!

The use of the safe period during the menopause is almost impossible because of the irregularity of the periods. Unless you are debarred by your religious beliefs from using any other method of birth control, or unless you don't mind the possibility of becoming pregnant, it would be better to forget the safe period altogether.

Sterilization

Sterilization for a man or woman is a possibility to be considered in careful consultation with a doctor. This method is very useful for those women who find they cannot use the pill or loop and are not very happy with other methods. Before sterilization is decided upon the doctor will discuss the operation fully with the couple, because once a man or woman has been sterilized it is very unlikely that the operation can be reversed.

Male sterilization, also known as vasectomy, is now becoming widely available. During the operation, the tiny tubes which carry the sperm are cut, under either a local or general anaesthetic in an outpatient clinic. It is important to remember that a man is not completely sterile until several months after the operation, because the sperm will not be immediately cleared from the tubes. Another form of birth control must be used until the doctor says the semen (the fluid released with the sperm during the climax) is completely free of sperm. Vasectomy makes no difference to a man's ability to have a climax and ejaculate.

When a woman is sterilized it is done under a general anaesthetic and means a small abdominal operation in hospital. The tubes from the ovaries to the uterus are cut and tied and she is sterile immediately. As both the ovaries are left a woman will continue her periods and go through the menopause in the usual way.

Sterilization is the most effective method of birth control if both the husband and wife are sure they do not want to have any more children. Anyone interested in sterilization must first consult their GP, who will then refer them to a consultant surgeon or to an FP Clinic. There is no physical reason whatsoever why sterilization should make any difference to anyone's sexual feelings. The simple tying and cutting of either the male or the female tubes in no way affects the production of sex hormones.

4. Health in middle age

The man or woman arriving at middle age does not have a blank sheet of paper on which to rewrite his or her health. How healthy you are at forty-five largely depends on decisions you took at ten, sixteen or twenty-five years of age. Decisions such as whether or not to smoke and drink, what was going to be your main social activity – pubs or a tennis court – and what job you were going to do.

How healthy you are at any stage of your life depends on:

1. Who your parents were, which means any family history of certain types of health problems such as varicose veins or sugar diabetes.

2. Your health in childhood. Children who suffer acute bronchitis may, as adults, be more likely to develop chronic bronchitis. If you had German measles as a child then you don't need to worry about German measles later on if you are pregnant. The wearing of ill-fitting shoes in childhood which harms the normal growth of the foot is often the reason for many of the foot troubles of later life such as bunions.

3. What sex you are. Obviously some health problems, especially those of the reproductive parts of the body, only apply to a man or a woman. But other conditions are more common in men, such as lung cancer because they smoke more (as female smoking increases, so have the numbers of women with lung cancer). More women than men are diagnosed as being depressed. The ratio is approximately 2 to 1. It has been suggested that in our culture women are more ready to admit their depression than men, who may think it is a sign of weakness to be depressed.

4. Whether you are sexually active or not. Most people during their life will form some sexual relationship unless, because of religious or social reasons, they have decided to remain chaste. Sexual activity is healthy and normal but it can have problems. A woman's first attack of cystitis (described in a later chapter) may be brought on by sexual activity. And of course VD can normally only spread by people changing sexual partners.

5. Whether or not a woman has been pregnant. Many of the so-called female problems were caused by difficult childbirth. Hopefully with our greatly improved maternity services these will disappear or become rare.

6. The job you do, and this includes the physically and mentally demanding job of being a wife and mother. Occupational medicine has established that various occupations have special risks, deep-sea diving and fishing have the highest death rates, businessmen are prone to over-eating and drinking, nurses to back injuries and psychiatrists to successful suicide.

7. Where you live. First of all, the kind of housing you have, is it warm, with a bathroom, toilet and hot water? How many people have to sleep in one room? Factors such as whether it is a flat, house or bed-sitting room in an inner city, suburb or country, noisy or quiet all affect the type of life that people can lead and their health. No wonder that people living on heavy lorry routes resort to using sleeping pills. Overcrowding helps the spread of infectious diseases. Another factor in where you live is the climate. Is it hot or cold? This affects the type of clothing you need, the kind of heating and sorts of exercise available. Skin cancer is very uncommon in the British Isles but far more common in people of British descent living in the sunny areas of South Africa, Australia and New Zealand where they are often sunburnt.

8. How much money you have and what you spend it on, especially food. The more money you have, the more able you are to spend money on a comfortable home, good food and sensible shoes, but it also means you can spend it on possible

health hazards such as too much drink, food and high living.
Affluence does not mean good health.

9. How willing you are to listen to advice and change your
way of life if you realize it is harmful.

So you enter middle age with many things written on your
health record and the most important thing is to take stock of
the situation and decide what are your good points and what
are problems. Once you know where you are, you can decide
what you want to do about it.

You might have a list like this:

age	47
sex	F
occupation	secretary/housewife, two children at home
weight	$\frac{1}{2}$ stone over recommended weight
smoking habit	4 a day
drink	rarely
exercise	walk around the park on Sundays
diet	*breakfast* coffee
	lunch sandwiches and cake
	dinner at home, three courses. Husband likes jam-roll puddings
	Biscuits and coffee through the day.
main problem	aching legs, swelling ankles in hot weather. Mother and grandmother had varicose veins. Often feels tired, but then finds it difficult to sleep at night

Or another list could be:

age	56
sex	M
occupation	carpenter and husband and father
weight	2 stone over recommended weight
smoking habit	50 a day

drink	2 pints of bitter with meal – goes drinking Friday and Saturday evening, at least 6–8 pints of beer
exercise	heavy work on building site, gardening at home
diet	*breakfast* cereal, cooked eggs and bacon, fried bread, toast, 3 teaspoons sugar in tea
	lunch sandwiches and flask of tea with plenty of sugar
	dinner always three course
main problem	shortness of breath, last winter off for 3 weeks with bad bronchitis

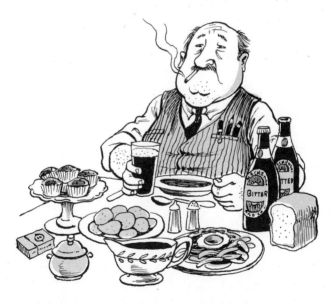

Both of these lists point to ways of life creating health problems. Without drastic changes, this man and woman could alter some of their habits so that within a few months they would feel fitter and healthier.

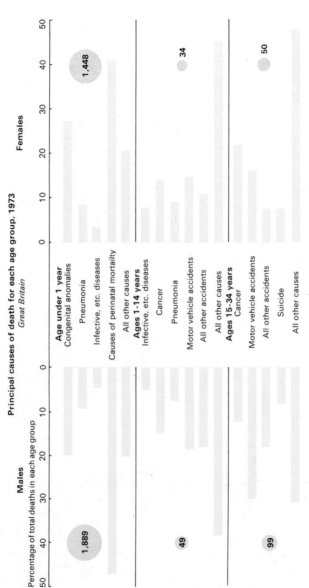

Principal causes of death for each age group, 1973

Great Britain

Males

Percentage of total deaths in each age group

Females

	Males	Females
Age under 1 year		
Congenital anomalies		
Pneumonia	1,889	1,448
Infective, etc. diseases		
Causes of perinatal mortality		
All other causes		
Ages 1–14 years		
Infective, etc. diseases		
Cancer		
Pneumonia	49	34
Motor vehicle accidents		
All other accidents		
All other causes		
Ages 15–34 years		
Cancer	99	50
Motor vehicle accidents		
All other accidents		
Suicide		
All other causes		

Figures in circles represent the death rate from *all* causes in 1973 per 100,000 population in each age and sex group.

Source: Office of Population Censuses and Surveys.

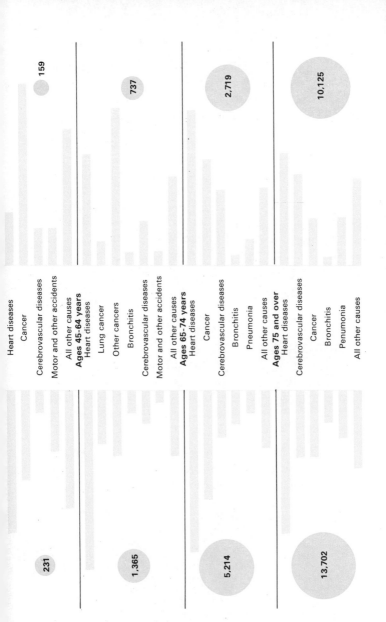

Heart diseases
Cancer
Cerebrovascular diseases
Motor and other accidents

Ages 45-64 years
Heart diseases
Lung cancer
Other cancers
Bronchitis
Cerebrovascular diseases
Motor and other accidents

Ages 65-74 years
Heart diseases
Cancer
Cerebrovascular diseases
Bronchitis
Pneumonia
All other causes

Ages 75 and over
Heart diseases
Cancer
Cerebrovascular diseases
Bronchitis
Penumonia
All other causes

All other causes

159

737

2,719

10,125

231

1,365

5,214

13,702

What would you recommend?

In Chapter 9 we will look at some ideas. See if yours are the same or if you have better ones.

What are the main health problems of middle age?

Well, apart from the conditions brought about by the menopause they tend to be conditions started at an earlier age, but now show themselves in a way that interferes with a person's life.

From this table of causes of death in various age groups you will see that around birth and the first year of life is quite dangerous. Once you get through that, you enter a safe period of life from one to thirty-five years, with accidents a main cause of death. After thirty-five the death rate starts to rise.

It is not the purpose of medical science to stop people from dying. We all must die, but it is the purpose of medical science to stop people dying unnecessarily at an early age or from suffering from a disease which prevents them being happy, useful members of a society.

That is why the rising death rate from thirty-five to seventy is so sad, because these are people dying too early; and when you look at the causes, heart disease, lung cancer, bronchitis, strokes, accidents, most could have been prevented.

The next chapters will now consider:

(a) health problems that don't threaten life
(b) male and female health problems
(c) life-threatening problems and what you can do about them
(d) psychological problems.

5. Health problems that don't threaten life

As we grow older our bodies start to show signs of the stress and strains and lack of attention that we have imposed on them. Often conditions that we put down to ageing are in fact caused by our way of life.

Hearing

Loss of hearing can be caused by being constantly in noisy atmospheres such as factories, or by living on noisy roads so that televisions and radios are turned up louder than normal. Employers are now realizing the danger of noise in the work place and supplying ear muffs where the noise level is above the safety limit. Other causes of loss of hearing are infections in the ear which could date back to childhood, and lastly excessive wax.

What to do

If you seem to be asking people to repeat themselves because you didn't hear them the first time or if your family moan about your lack of attention it could be that (a) you are not paying attention or (b) you have a loss of hearing.

1. Go to your doctor for a check-up. Any test and treatment would start from there. Don't ignore earache, or discharge from the ear hole, go to the doctor.

2. If you consider your work place to be very noisy, ask your union representative if any noise level tests have been carried out. If not, why not? The new 'Health and Safety at Work Act' makes the employers responsible for ensuring their

workers are in safe, healthy conditions and that the worker is responsible for using safety equipment, e.g. guards, ear muffs, that are provided.

3. If you don't have a union go to see the foreman, personnel officer or safety officer and ask to have noise level tests carried out.

4. The environmental health service is in charge of noise control. You will find them in the telephone book as a service of the local authority or Town Hall. Ask them for advice on noise control at work and at home. For example, if you live on a noisy road or near an airport you may be able to get a government grant for soundproofing your house.

If the noise level in our society, especially at the work place and in discotheques, were controlled, then many more people would have their hearing preserved into old age.

Sight

Our eyes do alter as we grow older. Most people who start to wear glasses or contact lenses as young people will go for regular check-ups, but the others often don't bother until headaches or blurring vision make them decide to ask the doctor to test their sight.

One of the common changes in sight is the need to hold a book further away while reading and needing a brighter light to read by comfortably. This reflects the change in the eye muscles.

Eyes that feel gritty and sore can occur at any age and red eyes, especially with a discharge, should be seen by a doctor.

A serious disease which can occur is glaucoma. There is normally fluid in the eyeball and this increases, causing pain, blurring of vision and lights with haloes around them. Don't ignore the symptoms, go to the doctor.

Seeing specks in front of your eyes is very common, especially when you are tired. It is caused by cells floating in the

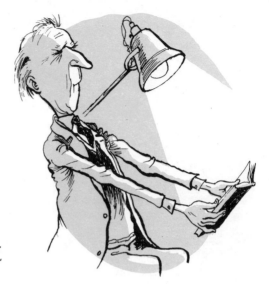

'Our eyes do alter
as we grow older'

fluid of the eye being reflected on to the part of the eye that sees. They can be annoying but they are not important.

Things to do

1. Make sure your eyes are well protected when you are doing jobs where there could be flying dust and chips.

2. If your job needs you to wear eye protection, wear it.

3. Keep your eyes clean. You don't need eye baths but make sure you wash your eyes thoroughly at least twice a day.

4. If you wear glasses or contact lenses then look after them. People are very careless with their glasses, putting them down so the lenses are scratched, never cleaning them and twisting the frames so the lenses are no longer set to give the proper vision.

5. Whether or not you wear glasses do have a periodic eye check up and don't ignore red, discharging eyes, pain, flashing lights, haloes around lights and blurring of your vision.

Teeth and gums

Dental decay is largely a problem of young people. Most people over twenty have fillings are having old fillings replaced, but it is the middle-aged who lose their teeth.

'Getting long in the tooth' is a common saying which many people believe is a natural process of ageing. It is not. You get long in the tooth because your gums are shrinking due to gum disease.

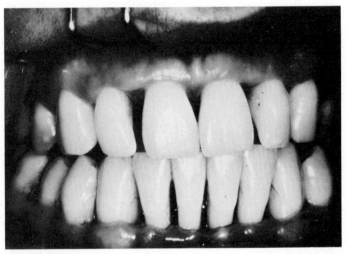

Gum disease

Run your tongue along your teeth. Do they feel furry? Or buy disclosing tablets from the chemist and suck one. Where your teeth are stained pink plaque is formed, a mixture of food and bacteria and acid. This causes infection of the gums – gingivitis.

> Do your gums ever bleed?
> Do any of your teeth sometimes feel loose?

If the answer is yes, you have gingivitis. If it is not stopped you will lose your teeth.

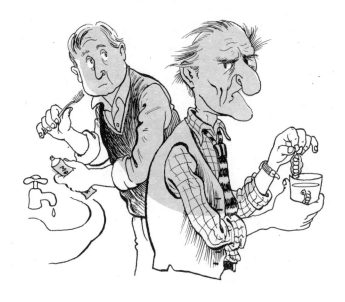

'So what,' you say, 'I can have false teeth fitted.' Which is quite true, but ask anyone with false teeth to answer truthfully which he or she would prefer.

What to do

1. It is amazing how many people who are very particular about being clean on the surface forget about their mouth. Thoroughly cleaning teeth and gums twice a day before or after eating is essential.

2. To see how well you clean your teeth, suck a disclosing tablet from the chemist or your dentist. This stains the plaque on your teeth. Try cleaning it off and this will give you an idea of the parts of your mouth you need to work hard on.

3. Ask your dentist to show you how to use dental floss and tooth picks to clean between your teeth.

4. Go for regular dental check-ups. If your dentist doesn't seem interested in prevention, ask him or her why.

5. Unfortunately the NHS doesn't pay your dentist for any time he spends on your dental health education. Maybe you could ask your MP why not.

6. Don't forget *you*, not your dentist, can save your teeth by restricting sugars and sweets, chewing chunky food and cleaning your teeth and gums thoroughly twice a day. You will be surprised how nice your mouth feels.

7. If you have dentures already remember your mouth alters in time and your dentures need checking to see they fit correctly. If your gums are sore go to the dentist, and remember to keep a healthy mouth you need clean dentures.

Skin

Most people are aware how marvellous their heart or brain are but don't think much of their skin except maybe women's faces and hands. We bake it in the sun, expose it to the cold, paint it with cosmetics, cover it with chemicals as we clean cars, baths, and other dirty jobs, cut and bruise it and take it for granted.

Our skin is a marvellous organ; it is protection, an elastic waterproof covering, it helps control our body temperature by sweating if we are hot and shivering if we are cold. It provides the sense of touch and can become tough and hard to protect those who do hard manual work.

As we grow older the skin becomes less elastic and drier, and it loses its thin fat layer. The more exposed the skin is to the sun, wind and rain, the faster this process becomes. Fine fair skins are affected faster than the more elastic oily dark skins which can take greater amounts of sunlight.

Wrinkles are a normal process and not a health problem. But middle age can bring skin problems. One common problem is acne rosea, a red rash, usually on the face. Another is a severe irritation of the skin between the legs in women. This can occur at any age but is particularly common during the menopause and is caused by the hormonal changes.

A possible distressing condition for women is the growth of facial hair. Just as their husbands may be bemoaning the loss of their hair due to changes in the male hormones, their wives may be developing facial hair due to their hormonal changes.

Because of the skin's constant exposure to chemicals of all kinds, men and women may develop contact dermatitis, a soreness of the skin due to a chemical. Many household products can cause this.

What to do

1. Keep the skin clean, especially skin folds such as armpits, under the breasts and between the legs. Piling talcum powder on to sweaty parts of the body creates mud, so remember to wash it off.

2. Washing removes the natural oils. Skin creams, however expensive and whatever the makers say they will do, can only soften and smooth the skin, preventing rapid fluid loss. Therefore skin creams are very useful for dry skin and preventing further fluid loss but they can't remove wrinkles.

3. If your hands are in water a lot use household gloves, and when using household cleaners read the instructions carefully.

4. If you don't want more than your share of wrinkles, protect your face and hands from the sun; but that means starting at twenty.

5. If you develop a rash or sore skin that doesn't clear in a couple of days, see your doctor.

6. If you do have tiny surface veins on your face, eating hot spicy food and drinking alcohol will make flushing of the face worse. So you have to decide which to give up.

Feet

Like our skin, our feet are an overlooked part of our bodies. We stuff them in the latest fashions regardless of what work we expect them to do. We never stretch or exercise them free

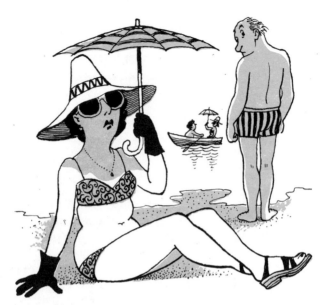

'Protect your face and hands from the sun'

of shoes and never really look at them. Then we wonder why they hurt.

Hard skin and corns are caused by too much pressure on one point over a period of time.

Bunions are caused by the big toe being pushed across to the other toes so that its big joint becomes swollen and sore.

As we grow older our feet often spread and we may need larger and wider shoes, yet how many people have their feet measured before they buy shoes or how many shops even offer that service?

What to do

1. Make sure your feet are clean and dry, especially between the toes, or painful infections such as athlete's foot will develop in the warm, damp space.

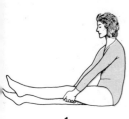

Foot exercises
1. Raise one leg, tightening your muscles
2. Point the foot down towards the floor
3. Turn your foot from side to side
4. Stretch your foot backwards and forwards
5. Rotate each foot ten times

1

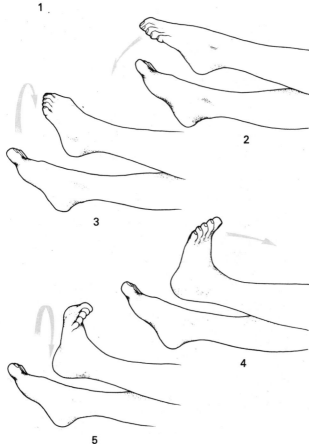

2

3

4

5

2. Prevent ingrowing toenails by cutting your nails straight across, not rounded.

3. Insist on having your feet measured when you buy shoes. If enough people did this the shops would be forced to provide a proper service.

4. Don't play around with your corns and hard skin but see a chiropodist who is specially trained in the care of feet.

5. If you have a bunion ask your doctor for advice; it may require an operation.

6. Do go barefooted at home. Get those shoes off and stretch those feet.

7. If you are overweight, lose it. Your feet will love you for it.

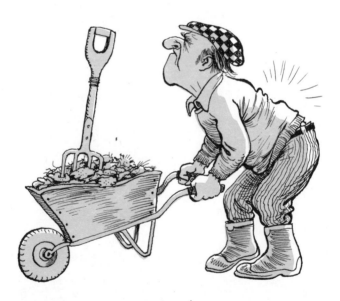

Back pain

Pain in the back, often called slipped disc, fibrositis, lumbago or sciatica, covers a multitude of conditions and causes. In 1971–2 in England and Wales 5 951 000 days of certified illness for men and 957000 days for women were recorded due to some type of back pain.

Occupations that involve lifting such as nursing, dockers and warehouse men are particularly prone.

What to do

1. If you have back pain now and then, think about what you have been doing. Are you driving long distances, have you been lifting heavy objects or carrying out heavy work you don't do normally? Have you got a new pair of shoes that are uncomfortable, particularly with high heels?

2. Bad posture can cause back pain and so can overweight.

3. Standing with your head up and shoulders back helps

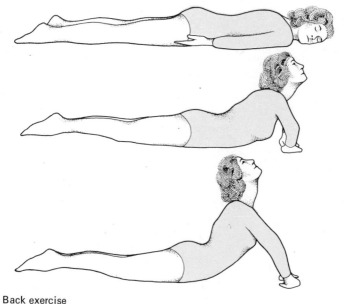

Back exercise
Starting from flat on the floor, slowly raise your head and shoulders.
Stop when you reach your comfortable limit and hold for five

balance you equally on your feet. High heels distort your posture.

4. To avoid straining your back, bend at the knees and use the strength of your legs to help you lift.

5. Strained backs are not always caused by lifting heavy objects. They might be quite light but you try to lift something while you are in an awkward position such as half turned.

6. Is your mattress firm? You don't have to rush out and spend hundreds of pounds on a special bed, but mattresses don't last for ever and sagging, lumpy mattresses don't help backs.

7. Do give your back some exercise.

8. If the pain persists or is sudden and sharp, see your doctor.

Varicose veins

This is a common condition of men and women but of course more obvious in women. Apart from the twisted veins which can be very unsightly, they cause the legs to ache and the ankles to swell, especially in hot weather and in jobs where you have to stand in one place for long periods. Very bad varicose veins can cause leg ulcers.

Varicose veins often run in families and are made worse by standing for long periods, lack of exercise, overweight and pregnancy. Blood returning to the heart from the feet has to come up against the force of gravity. Some veins can't cope and become varicosed.

Varicose veins are found not just in the legs but between the legs (these can be a problem in pregnancy) and around the opening of the back passage where they are called piles or haemorrhoids. These can become very painful and may bleed.

What to do

1. If you have a standing or sitting job, make sure you exercise the muscles in your legs, which helps the blood up.

You can do this by just moving up and down on your toes on one spot.

2. Get to enjoy a regular daily walk.

3. Wear support stockings. Don't be put off by the name; you can't see the difference, and what a support they are.

4. Do lie with your legs up for a few minutes each day to help return the flow of blood.

5. Do lose weight if you need to.

6. If you have piles don't become constipated (hard motions). Eating cereals like bran and wholemeal bread and drinking plenty of fluid is a help.

7. If in doubt do see your doctor, especially if you have piles that bleed or itch.

Cystitis

Cystitis is a feeling of burning discomfort when you pass water. You feel you want to go on passing water but only a little comes. Then two minutes later you want to go again. In a bad attack you may start to pass blood.

Cystitis is caused by inflammation (soreness and swelling) of the bladder and the passage leading from the bladder to the outside of the body (the urethra). It has many causes and it is not always a germ but can simply be bruising.

Cystitis is very common, especially in women who seem to develop it more readily than men. This is because of the way the female body is made. Therefore the comments for the rest of this section are about female cystitis but it should also be read by men as they can do a great deal to help prevent the problem for their partners.

You will see from the illustration overleaf that the opening of the back passage which is rich in germs is very close to the opening of the vagina and the urethra. Unlesss you are very careful in your personal hygiene like always cleaning yourself from front to back after a bowel motion or washing the area

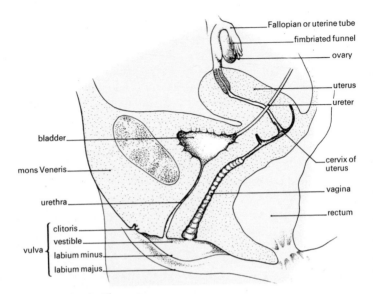

Female reproductive system

(and very few of us have bidets), you can see what a rich breeding ground for germs the area between the legs can be.

Also from the diagram you can see how close the vagina, bladder and urethra are. This is why cystitis is often associated with honeymoons and sexual intercourse. The delicate tissues of the urethra and bladder can be easily bruised unless the man is gentle in his love-making.

As has been pointed out already, the hormonal changes of the menopause can cause the vagina to become dry and less elastic, making intercourse difficult and painful. This could set off an attack of cystitis so that a woman who has never had the problem may develop it in middle years.

What you can do

1. Make sure your personal hygiene is excellent and the personal hygiene of your partner. You should always thorough-

ly wash with warm water before and after sexual intercourse. Warm or cool water is soothing if there is any bruising or discomfort.

2. Always make sure you empty your bladder completely when you pass water. So many people get careless in this rushing world and do not even allow time for the toilet. When you think you are finished, fold your arms across your tummy hard and push down. You might be surprised how much more you pass. Stale urine lying in the bladder is a breeding ground for germs. Make sure you tell your children to do it.

3. Always pass water before and as soon as possible after sexual intercourse.

4. If intercourse is uncomfortable try another position – the woman above the man, for example – and use a lubricant such as KY jelly, sold by all chemists.

5. 1 to 4 are sensible rules whether or not you have ever had cystitis. If you have an attack, as soon as you suspect something is wrong, e.g. your water stings when you pass it, start drinking at least half a pint every twenty minutes. Tea and coffee help you to pass water. Every hour for three hours take a level teaspoon of bicarbonate of soda in water. This will lessen the stinging feeling. Stay warm and wash yourself from back to front every time you go to the toilet.

6. If you have an attack of cystitis go to the doctor, but start your self help treatment at first sign.

7. There are so many sufferers of cystitis that there is now a club – the I & U Club. The address is at the back of the book.

6. Male and female health problems

MALE

Prostatectomy

More women than men suffer from cystitis but only men have a prostate gland which causes a very common problem of latter middle age, the constant desire to pass water, especially at night.

You will see that the prostate gland is around the urethra.

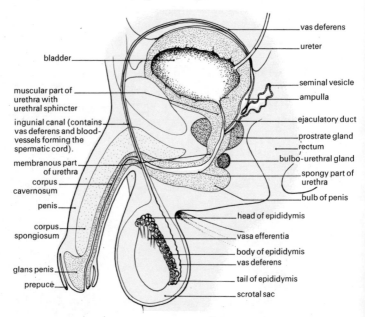

Male reproductive system

If this gland enlarges in size the tube becomes squeezed and the man will find it hard to empty his bladder completely.

The prostate gland enlarges for two reasons. Firstly and most commonly as a general ageing process, and secondly and less commonly as a cancerous growth. But it is one of the cancers which can be treated most successfully.

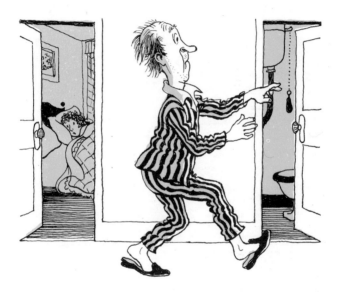

'A man may find himself getting up several times during the night'

What to do

1. Any man who has difficulty in passing water or who finds himself getting up several times during the night to pass water should go to his doctor. Of course if you drink several pints of beer or cups of tea before bed you will need to get up.

There is usually the feeling you want to pass more but it won't come.

2. The condition can be completely cured by an operation.

Impotence

Impotence can occur at any stage of a male's sexual life but can be a particular problem at middle age.

Fear of not being able to have an erection must be there in all men to a greater or lesser extent. Society sees it as a symbol of manhood.

As men reach middle age they are likely to have had the same sexual partner for quite a few years. Love-making may have settled down into an unexciting routine. Maybe you are both a bit overweight and feeling the years slipping by. As has been pointed out, men do not have a menopause but the male hormone testosterone does gradually decrease, in some men more rapidly than others.

Women are not always very easy people to live with during the menopause and there may be the added problem of teenage children finding their own feet as adults. Therefore the middle-aged man is in a challenging position sexually and it may be expressed as an increased sex drive outside home (the popular view) or a decreased interest.

Illness can dampen the sex drive and a man may wrongly believe that after a heart attack or his wife's hysterectomy a sexual life is no longer possible.

What to do

1. If you have a medical condition such as sugar diabetes or arthritis which seems to be affecting your sex drive, have a frank talk with your doctor. If you feel he or she would be unable to help (after all, few GPs are specially trained in sexual counselling) ask to see someone who specializes in these problems at the Family Planning Clinic or Marriage Guidance Council. You will find the number in the telephone book.

2. Do talk to your wife. Read a good sex manual together. Many women don't realize that they can stimulate their husbands by stroking and touching their bodies.

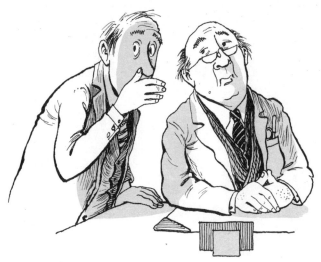

'Have a frank talk with your doctor'

3. Don't try to hurry things. If you have been ill your body needs time to repair itself.

4. *Don't bottle it up; seek help.*

FEMALE

Breasts

Breast cancer is one of the most treatable conditions, particularly if diagnosed early. Every woman, but especially those in middle age, should examine their breasts once a month between their periods. If your periods are finished then do it on the same date each month.

The drawings overleaf will show you how to do it.

If you feel a lump, go to your doctor. He or she will check it out for you.

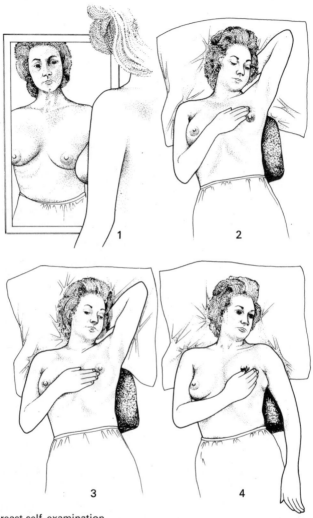

Breast self-examination
1. Look for any puckering or dimpling of the skin and any changes in the outline of your breasts
2–4. Lying down, with a towel under your back, using the flat of your fingers gently but firmly feel the breast. Divide the breast into four quarters and work in a circle around each one

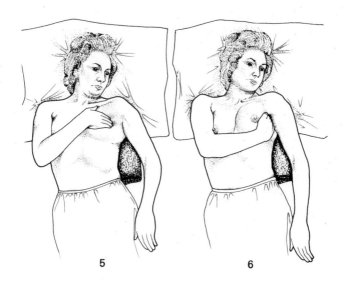

5. Feel around the nipple
6. Feel in the armpit
Moving the towel to the other side, repeat with the other breast

Cervix

The cervix is the part of the womb that is at the top of the vagina. (See diagram on page 64.)

This is another area like the breasts where women do develop cancer but where it can be easily found by a cyto test, which should be done at least once a year if you are over thirty-five. This is a simple vaginal examination, familiar to those of you who have had babies. A few cells are painlessly taken from the cervix. They are looked at under a microscope and the doctor can tell if any of them are likely to develop into cancerous cells.

Most women's tests show healthy cells. If there is a query she would be taken into hospital for further tests and treatment.

Hysterectomy

A hysterectomy is the removal of the womb and sometimes the ovaries. If the ovaries are removed it means the woman loses her supply of female hormones, so these must be replaced by hormones in tablet form.

Hysterectomies are usually done if the woman has bad fibroids, spongy growths on the wall of the womb so that she loses a lot of blood, or less commonly for cancer.

Unusual bleeding from the vagina should always be reported to the doctor, but women during the menopause may find it difficult to decide what is unusual bleeding.

You should report:

1. Flooding – large amounts of blood at the expected time of the period or at any other time.

2. Spotting – small drops of blood on your pants on and off through the month.

3. An unexpected bleeding some time after your periods have appeared to finish.

Hysterectomy is a special operation for many women and it must be stressed that losing a uterus does not make you less of a woman.

The vagina is left and once the woman is healed there is no reason why sexual relationships should not recommence, gently and with care at first, and be as good as ever.

If you do have a hysterectomy and you have an active sex life, make sure your surgeon discusses it with you. If he or she doesn't mention it, you do. They will be the best people to advise on your post-operation return to health.

Repair operation

In some women the muscles which hold the womb, vagina, bladder, and back passage in place become weaker. This can be a problem for women who had difficult labours and who either were not taught or didn't do their post natal excercises. The first sign might be that when you laugh or cough to your horror you wet your pants.

What to do

1. You can work on those muscles to strengthen them. Make sure you never let your bladder get over full. Being overweight doesn't help.

2. Lie on the floor, cross your ankles and pull hard to tighten the muscles between your legs.

3. Do this every day for a week. At the end of the week, do your muscles feel stronger?

4. If you can get no movement from your muscles and you find it difficult to hold your water, go to your doctor.

5. If he or she considers it necessary, there is an operation which tightens up the muscles.

6. All women should regularly practise tightening the muscles between the legs. Not only does it improve their health and prevent weak bladders but it can improve their sexual responses.

Vaginal discharges

Like cystitis, these are very common but only in recent years have people started to talk about them. The most common is thrush and the second condition is trichomoniasis.

There is always a slight normal discharge from the vagina. But a thick white or yellow discharge that causes irritation and soreness is not normal.

What to do

1. Follow the personal hygiene advice given for cystitis.

2. Wear cotton pants (nylon causes sweating which makes

it worse). Change your pants once or more a day and wash them in very hot water.

3. Go to your doctor. Both these conditions can be cured but do reoccur, so make sure you go on with strict personal hygiene and encourage your husband to do the same.

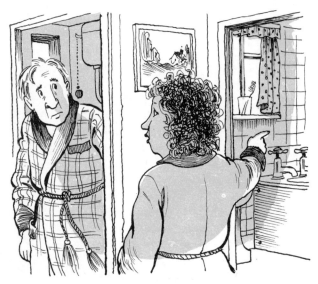

'Encourage your husband to do the same'

4. Men can develop thrush, so if you have had it make sure he has a check as well.

5. These are not venereal diseases but they are conditions which are often treated at special clinics which specialize nowadays in a wide range of conditions related to the bladder and reproductive system of men and women. They will see you without a note from your doctor, and you find the address and number of your closest clinic in the telephone book.

7. Life-threatening conditions

It has been said that if we exercised a bit more self control over how much we ate, drank, and smoked, took a walk every day and learnt to relax rather than tying ourselves up in knots of fury, more lives could be saved than by all the expensive pills and machines that we call medicine.

Our society has got the idea that it is doctors who make us healthy. It is not. Doctors treat us when we are ill and except for the few thousands of doctors and nurses in public health most of the National Health Service patches up people after the damage is done.

What keeps us healthy: our clean water and sewage disposal, control of food hygiene, pollution control, a balanced diet, regular exercise and rest, our personal hygiene and our bodies' defences against disease helped by immunization.

Clean water and food, sewage and pollution control are community responsibilities; the rest is up to us.

When you look at the main killers of middle age – heart and circulation conditions, bronchitis and lung cancer and accidents – they are all related to the way we live. As the factors in all these conditions are so closely related, this section is divided into the conditions and then what we can do.

Heart and circulatory conditions

The heart is a very strong organ of the body beating at sixty to eighty times a minute (much faster in stress) from birth to death. (Before birth the heart beats faster.)

It is divided into four chambers, the right two separated from the left two. The right side collects blood from the veins and sends it through the lungs. The left side then sends the oxygen-rich blood through the arteries to all parts of the body.

Blood pressure is the force at which the blood is pumped out into the arteries.

With a blood pressure of $\frac{120}{80}$, 120 is the pressure at which the blood is forced out of the heart. 80 is the pressure in the artery while the heart is at rest.

A blood pressure of $\frac{160}{100}$ shows that while the heart has to use a high pressure to send the blood out, the heart does get a rest.

A blood pressure of $\frac{160}{140}$ shows the heart is resting at a high pressure.

This sort of high blood pressure is a strain on the heart muscle.

High blood pressure can run in families but is closely associated with stress, overweight and lack of exercise, but there can be other less obvious causes which are difficult to establish.

Coronary artery disease is when porridge-like material starts to form on the walls of arteries. This makes the artery smaller so the blood has difficulty in flowing through. This is associated with a diet high in animal fats, e.g. butter, lack of exercise and smoking.

Angina pectoris is often just called angina. It is a pain caused by the heart muscles being starved of oxygen so that they get cramp. The pain can be heavy across the chest, running down the left arm or up into the neck and face. It might be felt as shoulder tip pain, and is often mistaken for indigestion. Rest eases the pain.

It must be reported to a doctor

Coronary thrombosis is a clot of blood in the arteries of the heart. If we cut ourselves, unless it is a major blood vessel we don't bleed to death because our blood can thicken, forming a clot. But if these clots form in an artery they are carried along, and as the artery narrows the clot will eventually block it. Clots can form in the veins especially of the leg, blocking a leg vein (venous thrombosis) or clots can form in lungs or in the brain. Clots in the brain are the cause of strokes.

Coronary thrombosis causes a gripping severe pain in the chest and often down the arm and into the neck. It is not stopped by rest. *The patient should be placed in a sitting position and a doctor called immediately.*

Respiratory conditions

Bronchitis has its beginnings in childhood infections, air pollution, the damp climate and smoking. The tubes leading to the lungs become irritated and thick mucus forms which is an ideal breeding ground for germs. Breathing becomes difficult. Chronic (long-term) bronchitis is a major cause of lost work-time in Britain.

Lung cancer is a major cause of death of middle-aged men and, as women's smoking increases, of women. The lung cancer associated with smoking is one of the most preventable of all diseases. There is a type of lung cancer which non-smokers develop but it is rare. There are very few doctors who do not accept the evidence of the close connection between smoking and lung cancer and other cancers such as that of the bladder.

Accidents

Accidents so often could have been prevented if only someone had followed the rules or used their common sense. Middle-

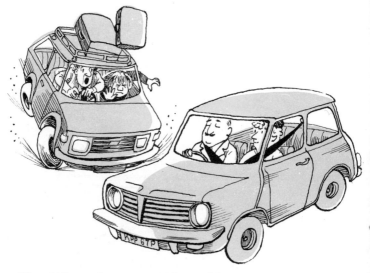

'The middle-aged can set a good example'

aged people are less accident prone than the very young or the very old. The new regulations about wearing seat belts should improve the accidents statistics and the middle-aged can set a good example to the others by making sure they wear their belts.

Associated problems

Associated with life-threatening conditions are other problems which often are important factors in how well a person survives a life-threatening condition.

Sugar diabetes or diabetes mellitus often shows up in middle age in a routine urine test or with symptoms of tiredness or an attack of thrush. In middle age (as opposed to it starting in childhood) it is associated with overweight and a diet high in refined sugars and that includes alcohol. Diet will usually control the condition in middle age.

Digestive problems such as wind or constipation may develop in middle age. Is it a particular food that brings on wind, such as cabbage or brussels sprouts? Eating rapidly does not help. Constipation can be relieved without pills by drinking more fluid and increasing fibre – bran, wholemeal bread and fruit and vegetables.

Ulcers are more common in men than women and appear usually from thirty onwards. If you have pain before meals which is relieved by food, especially bland food and milk, do not just take anti-acid tablets; go and see your doctor.

Gall bladder trouble is more common in women and seems to affect the overweight more than the thin and active. Remember the rhyme 'Fair, Fat and Forty Female' as a description of the typical gall bladder patient. It shows as discomfort after eating, tenderness below the ribs and pain in the shoulder. In bad cases the patient may look yellow – jaundice. You need to consult a doctor. Diet may control the situation but often an operation is needed to remove the gall stones.

Alcoholism   Dependence on alcohol in both men and women is a largely ignored health problem in our society especially among the middle-aged.

Heavy drinking does not mean a person is an alcoholic but it will certainly add to any weight problems.

A true alcoholic cannot do without a drink but will frequently go to great lengths to hide the fact of his drinking. Marital stress, problems at work and money problems are common complications. Alcoholism is an illness and the alcoholic needs support and understanding, not rejection, as does his family.

The family doctor should be the first contact for help but there are specialized organizations such as Alcoholics Anonymous who will help.

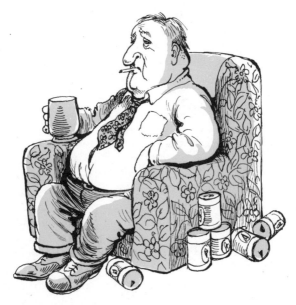

'Heavy drinking . . . will certainly add to any weight problems'

Signs you should watch for and act on

The body has devised its own warning system of problems and it is worthwhile remembering them.

Don't ignore indigestion. It might not be your stomach but your heart.

Lumps in any part of the body, especially if they seem to get bigger, need to be examined. Most of them are harmless but it is best to be sure.

Unusual bleeding, especially continuous and heavier than a normal period, and blood in the urine or stools should be reported. Black, shiny stools can be a sign of bleeding.

A great many people suffer needlessly for years with bleeding piles. A simple operation will solve the agony and may also prevent anaemia caused by the years of constant loss of blood.

A persistent cough, especially if you cough up phlegm and blood, needs attention. If you smoke, all the more reason to stop. Smoking only aggravates the condition.

Sores which do not heal and loss of weight without design should not be ignored. Neither should persistent hoarseness and changes in bowel or bladder habit. Of course, holidays, especially abroad, or a change of life-style like a new job or home may lead to a temporary change in bowel habits, but if it persists see your doctor.

8. Psychological problems

Medical science tends to put health problems in little boxes.

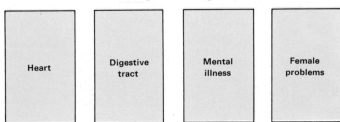

| Heart | Digestive tract | Mental illness | Female problems |

It is much easier to understand things this way, but it is not a true picture of life. A man may have a heart attack at forty-five. He may be overweight, smoking a lot and drinking a lot. Why? Because he is worried he might lose his job. His wife, now the children have grown up, has trained as a teacher and now has a world of her own quite different to his. And to crown it all his mother, whom he loved dearly, died six months ago.

Hospitals know how to treat people with heart attacks; they can give people drugs, diet sheets and advise them to give up smoking and moderate their drinking. What they are not very good at is helping people with all the other problems which probably made them ill in the first place.

Depression

This is particularly true of the biggest psychological problem of middle age – depression. In 1972, 23 406 people were treated for depression, 16 206 women and 7200 men. These figures represent the tip of an iceberg. In a report of the Royal College of General Practitioners in 1972 they estimate that 200 of all the cases that each GP saw in a year were for emotional reasons. Everyone becomes depressed at times – that is natural. When it interferes with the person's ability to carry on a normal life, depression is an illness, but so often the sufferer is greeted with 'Pull yourself together'. At times we do need to be told that, but not someone with depression.

Signs of clinical depression are:

1. Loss of appetite, although some people just eat and eat for comfort, not because they are hungry.

2. Difficulty in sleeping.

3. Feelings of anxiety. All of us feel anxious at times, but in depression the anxiety develops over things which were once no bother like buying a new dress or going to work.

4. Feelings of worthlessness and becoming over self-critical.

5. Excessive tiredness, lack of sex drive and in men impotence may develop.

6. In deep depression thoughts of suicide may develop.

7. Some depressive illnesses go through manic phases when the person is cheerful, prepared to change the world and seems to have boundless energy. This can quickly change back to the depressive state.

8. Depression is not a modern disease. Melancholia has long been described by writers and poets. Many of our most creative artists have suffered from it.

9. It can be successfully treated but it can recur.

There are wide varieties of opinion on the cause and treatment of depression. Some would argue that it is the social conditions that start it off and the treatment should be the social conditions not drug therapy. Others would say personality type is a factor and others that drug therapy is efficient and safe.

What is safe to say is:

1. Depression is an illness and medical help should be sought by either the sufferer or the family.

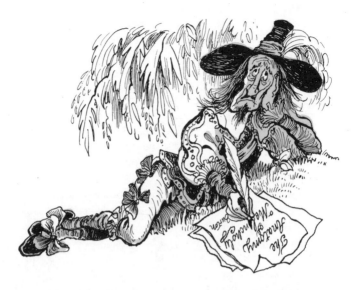

'Melancholia has long been described by writers and poets'

2. If social conditions, loss of job or partner, or bad housing do seem to be important factors then drug therapy alone will only dampen the condition, not cure it. The social conditions must be tackled.

3. Anyone suffering from depression and their family and friends need to explore why did this happen and can we by the way we act to one another stop it happening again or lessen the effect.

4. Our society needs more provision of good community care of people who are or have been mentally ill. It needs employers, personnel officers and workmates who will be understanding and helpful. You may never have been depressed but what about your reactions to other people. Are you sympathetic?

5. MIND is an organization which exists to promote good

mental health. It is an active pressure group for better services and prevention of mental illness. It needs enthusiastic people like you to get involved. Their address is in the back of the book.

Grief

It might seem strange to include grief in this section but grief is one of the most ignored human emotions in present-day Western society. It wasn't always, and in many societies today the public display of grief and mourning is considered natural. Many psychologists believe that our bottling up of grief is a cause of many problems including depression and accidents.

Grief is an emotion like love which can only really be understood by those who have experienced it.

The entry into middle age might also be marked by the first loss of a parent, spouse or close friend. Some people describe the overwhelming sense of loss as a sorrowing not for the person who is dead but for themselves who are left behind. People who believed that they had prepared themselves well for the death of a loved one express surprise at the overwhelming emotion they felt; and that they have no one to share it with; that other people become embarrassed and want to avoid talking about the person who has died, not through unkindness but because they don't know how to handle the situation.

Death has become a taboo subject in our society in place of sex. Yet we all must die and face death in our family and friends. There is no need to return to the elaborate rituals of Victorian death but we do need to recognize that grief is a natural human emotion that must be allowed to run its course. Tears in a man or woman should not be seen as a shameful weakness but a natural healing outlet.

So don't let us feel embarrassed but let us welcome grief when it comes as a sign of a healthy natural emotion.

An important point to make: it is not unusual for someone

who has suffered grief, the loss of a spouse, parent, child or close friend to suffer an accident themselves in the months following the loss. Maybe its because grief interferes with our normal life-protecting responses which so often save us from accidental injury.

9. Now for the good news

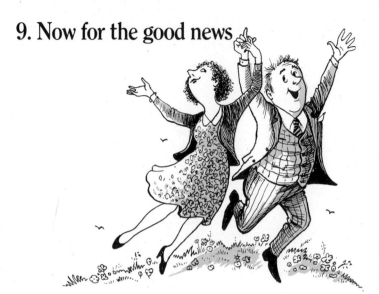

By now you are probably thinking that middle age is all doom and gloom so let's forget it anyway. Well, in case you didn't notice, in nearly all the problems was the suggestion that you could by your own actions either prevent them or do something about them.

So here are some positive suggestions.

How's your weight?

From the tables on the following page, are your normal, over or underweight?

Normal – congratulations; just make sure you stay that way.

Underweight – ask the question why. Have you been losing weight latterly without trying? Or have you been dieting too hard? Stress and worry can cause lack of appetite. If that seems to be the reason, can you alter the situation? Have a word with your doctor. He can recommend the foods to help you put on weight like cakes, potatoes and fresh bread.

Men

Add 7lb. for clothes and 1 in. for shoes	ft.	in.	ideal weight range lb.	lb.	lb.		overweight range lb.	very overweight range
	5	1	105	117	128	to	140	and over
	5	2	108	120	132	to	144	and over
	5	3	111	123	135	to	148	and over
	5	4	113	126	139	to	151	and over
	5	5	117	130	142	to	155	and over
	5	6	120	134	145	to	160	and over
	5	7	124	138	152	to	166	and over
	5	8	128	142	156	to	170	and over
	5	9	131	146	161	to	175	and over
	5	10	135	151	166	to	181	and over
	5	11	140	155	171	to	186	and over
	6	0	144	160	175	to	191	and over
	6	1	148	164	180	to	197	and over
	6	2	152	169	186	to	203	and over
height without shoes	6	3	157	174	191	to	209	and over

Women

Add 5lb. for clothes and 1 in. for shoes	ft.	in.	ideal weight range lb.	lb.	lb.		overweight range lb.	very overweight range
	4	8	87	97	106	to	116	and over
	4	9	89	99	109	to	119	and over
	4	10	92	102	112	to	122	and over
	4	11	95	105	116	to	126	and over
	5	0	97	108	119	to	130	and over
	5	1	100	111	122	to	133	and over
	5	2	103	115	126	to	137	and over
	5	3	106	118	130	to	142	and over
	5	4	110	123	135	to	147	and over
	5	5	114	127	139	to	152	and over
	5	6	117	131	144	to	157	and over
	5	7	121	135	148	to	161	and over
	5	8	125	139	152	to	166	and over
	5	9	128	143	157	to	171	and over
height without shoes	5	10	132	147	161	to	176	and over

Weight tables

Overweight – and lots of us are. Well, there is good news for you: everybody can lose weight. Don't say you have tried every method and it has failed. You too can lose weight once you find a method you are happy with and will stick to. There is no magic, only will-power and perseverance.

Anyone who has been overweight for years should check with their doctor before starting a diet. Some hospitals do now run Obesity Clinics that specialize in people with special weight problems. We eat food to provide us with energy to live and work. Any food that we eat more than is needed for that day's work gets stored as fat for the lean months. But the lean months rarely come in our society. The amount of energy we need to do a job is measured in calories. Food has been analysed to give its calorie value. For example, three teaspoons of boiled potato is eighty calories.

A moderately active middle-aged man needs 2500 to 3500 calories a day and a woman between 2000 and 3000. To lose weight you need to eat fewer calories than your calorie-needs a day. That way your body will start to burn up fat.

However you decide to work out what foods you will eat, basically to lose weight you must eat fewer calories than you use up in work and movement.

So a typist should aim for about 1000 calories and a heavy manual worker 2000. Slimming machines, massage, etc., may make you feel better but they cannot get rid of fat. Only the body burning it up will.

How to diet

1. It depends on what sort of person you are. Some people like to go it alone and, with a book of calorie values for food, succeed by themselves.
2. Others need support. There are now plenty of slimming clubs and magazines to provide help and support of others with the same problems. Some methods concentrate on calorie

control, others on avoiding or limiting certain foods. You may need to try several to find the way that suits you.

3. Slimming clubs do cater for men.

4. Do enlist the help of your friends and family. Those thoughtless people who tempt the dieter from his or her good resolves are not acting as true friends.

5. Food is an important social activity in our society. A good cook is admired. See if your cooking skills can be turned to the production of low calorie masterpieces.

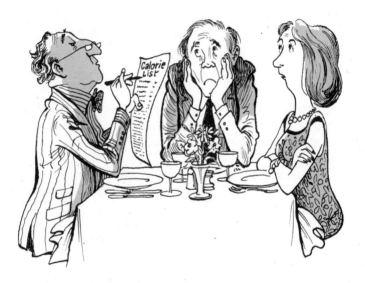

6. Don't become a calorie-counting bore. It's a good way to lose friends.

7. Do buy a piece of clothing you really like in a size smaller than you are. Use that as your reward for being good, not a cream bun.

8. Once you have gained your desired weight your appetite should have adjusted itself to your new level of food intake. Now it is a matter of watching yourself to make sure bad old habits don't creep back.

Every time you feel the old urge for some rich and stodgy food, just look in the mirror, if you can, at the new slim you.

Smoking

It is often said that health education is all about urging people to give up things they like such as food, booze, smokes and sex. 'Where would be the excitement in life if we gave up our little treats?' is the cry.

Health from this point of view is presented as dull and unexciting. Well, it depends on who you want to fool, yourself or others. When did you last think a breathless, red-faced, nicotine-stained, boozy man or woman an exciting, thrilling life and soul of the party?

Apart from the health hazard, smoking is at last being recognized as the anti-social habit it really is. Compare the state of a smoking compartment of a train, bus or tube to the non-smoking one. And someone has to clean that up. How many miles of valuable forest and wild life have been lost due to careless smokers?

And the argument 'it only affects me' doesn't work any more now we know the effect that mothers smoking in pregnancy can have on their unborn babies and that non-smokers sitting with smokers are forced to breathe polluted air and also absorb nicotine.

But you can give up, and here are some suggestions:

1. Decide two or three weeks in advance that you're going to quit. Cut down your smoking gradually over the three weeks. And then stop for good.

2. Many smokers find it easier to give up while they're on holiday. This applies especially to habitual smokers. The change in their day-to-day habits helps them break the smoking habit. If you're not going on holiday for some time, it may work if you alter your everyday routine. Walk to work for a change. Sit in a different chair. Read another daily newspaper.

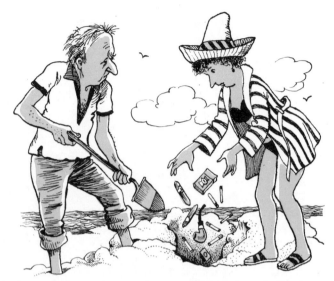

'Many smokers find it easier to give up while they're on holiday'

3. Change your eating habits. For some reason eating seems to trigger the craving for a cigarette. There's probably no physical explanation. More likely, smokers habitually light up after a meal, a snack or with a cup of tea or a pint of beer. For the first few days try and do without all drinks and snacks that you would normally follow with a cigarette. And make a really conscious effort not to smoke after meals.

(Incidentally, if you put on a few pounds when you give up smoking, don't worry. This is easy to control by a little careful attention to diet.)

Exercise

I expect by now you are asking where is the good news? Can exercise be good news? Well, if you have visions of large muscular men heaving shot puts or lifting weights, or drill sergeants you hated, or falling flat on your face after being made to jump over a jumping horse, I don't blame you for being put off. But, exercise can be F U N.

We have lost the sheer pleasure of enjoying our bodies' movement, and for this about half of the blame must go to the old-fashioned drill way that sport was once taught in schools. Luckily that is now changing.

It doesn't matter what the exercise is as long as you *enjoy* it.

When did you last feel really physically tired, a satisfying feeling?

With exercise comes relaxation. So many people cannot sleep at night because although they are mentally tired their bodies are tensed and tight. Tonight when you go to bed, see how you are lying; are your hands gripped tight? Then lie on your back, consciously tighten all your muscles and then let go, letting out a deep breath. See if you feel different.

It is no use forcing yourself into a set of exercises you hate because you won't keep it up. Whatever you choose to do, it must fit in with your everyday life.

Here are a few suggestions:

1. Get off the bus or tube two stops before work and walk. This is only enjoyable if your walking route is away from heavy traffic.

2. If you like dogs but haven't one, offer to walk an elderly neighbour's dog after dinner each night. It will do both of you good.

3. Work out a set of exercises you enjoy and do them daily. There are some suggestions at the end.

4. Join a club, for example badminton, golf, rambling, bowling, learn to swim at your local pool. You are never too old.

5. If your local roads are not infested with heavy lorries, buy a second-hand bike for local excursions and save on bus fares and petrol.

6. Many local authorities run keep-fit classes. Suggest to

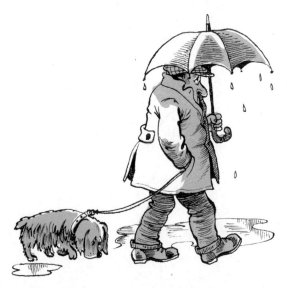

'Offer to walk an elderly neighbour's dog after dinner each night. It will do both of you good'

your personnel officer, if you have one, that your firm might start a keep fit class.

7. Have you ever thought of yoga or meditation? Classes and clubs are often run by adult education services or by interested groups who might advertise in the local press.

8. Remember it doesn't matter how unfit you are, you can be better than you are. Don't rush it. Take it stage by stage and you will be surprised how quickly you will feel better and look better.

Middle age doesn't need to be the start of a slow or rapid decline into indifferent health and a few interests, but the opportunity for new activities, and great enjoyment of life with a fit and healthy body.

Remember:

1. A balanced sensible diet.
2. No smoking and if you drink, drink in moderation.

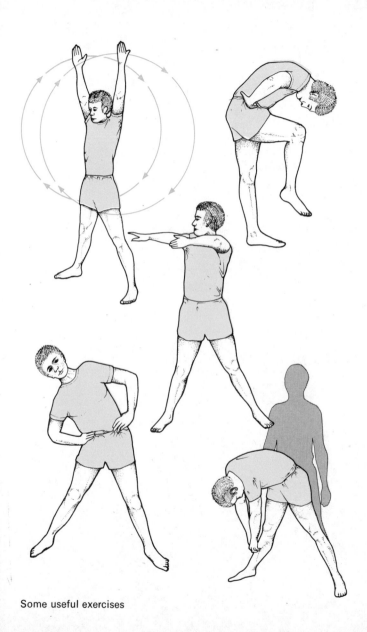

Some useful exercises

3. Regular enjoyable exercise.
4. Relaxation.
5. Treasure your family and friends – you need to work to make relationships that are worthwhile.

Conclusion

In Chapter 4 we looked at two possible lists that a middle-aged man and woman might make about their health.

By now you will know what changes they need to make you feel fit.

The woman only needs to lose a small amount of weight and, by changing her lunch from sandwiches and cake to a small salad and low calorie squash, not having biscuits with her coffee and persuading her husband to have fresh fruit for dessert rather than jam rolls, she should be able to lose weight. She only smokes four cigarettes a day so she should be able to give them up with no trouble. Her walk around the park could be supplemented by ten minutes' exercise a day ending up with her legs raised above her head and then relaxation. The exercise, and wearing support stockings, should help her varicose veins and swelling ankles and the relaxation her ability to sleep at night.

The man has a more difficult problem. He has a heavy job and is still overweight. If he doesn't do something soon he will not be able to go on working on a building site and therefore would have to take lighter work with loss of earnings.

He must give up smoking if he is not to develop long-term bronchitis. He must lose weight. If he cuts down on his beer, sugar in his tea and fried bread at breakfast, that alone could make a big difference to his calorie intake.

Research has shown that wives are the most important influence on how seriously a man takes his health, so his wife must be involved.

He already does quite a lot of exercise but maybe he could take up a sport like bowling which would give an added

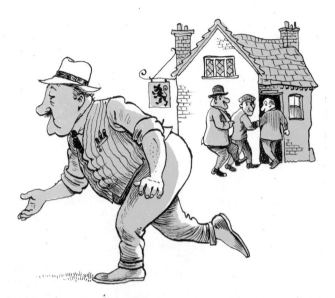

'Bowling might take the social place of the regular drinking evenings'

interest and maybe take the social place of the regular drinking evenings. It doesn't mean he has to forgo the pub if he is strong enough to control the amount of beer that he drinks and ignore the cigarettes. He is giving up something but he is getting something back in return – health.

Middle age is a time for challenge and adventure. We are always trying to find out who we are, what are we and what is the purpose of life? But at least by middle age we are probably clearer as to how well we can answer these questions than we were when we were young.

Accepting what we can do does not have to be giving in, but knowing our strengths and weaknesses and concentrating on what we can do well.

Children leaving home can mean time for you to develop your own interests.

Redundancy, although traumatic, could also be the chance to retrain for something you never thought you would get the chance to do.

Many people now in middle age missed out on their education because of the war and other social conditions. Many colleges, polytechnics, extra-mural departments of universities and the Open University provide opportunities for a second chance at an education.

The Department of Employment also runs a career guidance service for people who want to retrain or change work direction New towns may be a chance for a new job and new housing.

The middle years are also a time for both men and women to prepare for the time when they no longer have to work. Most people consider the financial preparation needed for retirement, but now is the time to develop those interests which make all the difference between a happy contented retirement and empty time-hanging years.

How people adapt to middle age depends on their background, their state of health and what is happening at that time in their life. The old cliché 'you are only as old as you feel' has a great deal of truth in it. No one can control all the circumstances of his or her life, but it is possible with practice to learn to step outside oneself for a minute and try to see things as an outside person would. It often helps.

Most people sail through the middle years, dealing with the occasional crisis and finding contentment in the fact that they have come to terms with themselves and their life. Everybody has minor problems and we hope this book may have helped with some of them. Others have problems too large to carry by themselves and it is hoped that they are reassured that help is available if they will seek it.

List of addresses of useful organisations

Abortion

If you suspect an unwanted pregnancy you can see your doctor or your local Family Planning Clinic. If you decide that an abortion is the right solution they can refer you to the local hospital.

If you want to consult a private organization the following have a high reputation for professional service.

Pregnancy Advisory Service Ltd
40 Margaret Street
London W1

British Pregnancy Advisory Service
1st Floor, Guildhall Buildings
Navigation Street
Birmingham B2 487

Alcoholism

You could see your own doctor but if you need the help of others with the same problem then

Alcoholics Anonymous
11 Redcliffe Gardens
London SW10

will help.

Their aim is to stay sober and help other alcoholics achieve sobriety. They would also provide local addresses.

Other organizations are:

Alcoholics Recovery Project
25 Camberwell Grove
London SE5

National Council of Alcoholism
45 Great Peter Street
London SW1

Alcoholism Information Centre
25A Wincott Street
London SE11

Birth control and family planning

Birth control and family planning also include advice on sub-fertility and genetic counselling which could be very important for a middle-aged couple thinking about having a baby.

Most GPs now provide a family planning service but you will need to be referred to a specialist clinic for sub-fertility or genetic counselling.

You can also attend your local Family Planning Clinic without going through your doctor. Their addresses are in your local telephone book. Family planning is free on the NHS.

If you want specialized help you could contact

The Family.Planning Association
27–35 Mortimer Street
London W1N 8BQ

Cystitis

See your own doctor. The Health Education Council produces a leaflet on self-help for cystitis which your doctor may have or you could ask at your local health district office. You can also contact the

U & I Club
Secretary: Mrs Kilmartin
9E Compton Road
London N1

Health services

The GP is the main point of reference to specialized aspects of the health services but Family Planning Clinics, Well Women Clinics for the cyto test and special clinics for VD are all available without reference from your doctor.

Legal advice

Most solicitors provide a legal aid scheme under which people on restricted incomes can get legal advice at reduced rates. A pamphlet called *Legal Aid and Advice: How to obtain the Help of a Lawyer* can be obtained from

> The Law Society
> 113 Chancery Lane
> London WC2A 1PL

Local authority education services

Your local education office should be able to tell you about courses and grants for mature students. They will also have lists of all adult education courses, both day and evening, in your area.

Under the government retraining scheme the Department of Employment runs the TOPS grant scheme. Your local employment office has details of the scheme and of the courses available, which range from typing to professional training. Local libraries also keep information on courses and training.

Local authority social services

Your local offices should be able to advise you about exactly what services are provided as they do vary slightly from area to area but they will include all social workers, home help services, community care of the mentally ill, laundry services, day nurseries, fostering and adoption, aids for the disabled and meals on wheels.

The *Sunday Times* have published a *Self Help Directory*, edited by Judith Chisholm and Oliver Gillie which contains a wider range of organizations than is possible in this book. You could also consult the *Guide to the Social Services, 1976*, published by Macdonald & Evans in association with the Family Welfare Association.

The menopause

The National Health Service does have a number of Menopause and Well Women Clinics to provide specialized advice and treatment for women during the menopause. Telephone your local health district office for information on what is provided locally as there may be a new clinic set up in your area that is not on the following list of established Menopause Clinics.

Aberdeen: Gynaecology Endocrine Clinic, Dept of Obstetrics and Gynaecology, Aberdeen University, Foresthill.

Barnet (Herts): Family Centre, Wood Street.

Belfast: Samaritan Hospital, Lisburn Road.

Birmingham: The Menopause Clinic, Professorial Unit, Women's Hospital, Showell Green Lane, Sparkhill.

   also: Dudley Road Hospital, Dept of Obstetrics and Gynaecology, Birmingham 18.

   also: St Chads' Hospital, Hagley Road, Edgbaston.

Brighton: The Menopause Clinic, Dept of Obstetrics and Gynaecology, Royal Sussex Hospital.

Bristol: Menopause Clinic, South Mead Hospital, Westbury-on-Trim.

Durham: Menopause Clinic, Dept of Gynaecology, Dryburn Hospital.

Edinburgh: Gynaecological Out-Patients, Royal Infirmary, Dept of Obstetrics and Gynaecology, 39 Chalmers Street, Edinburgh, EH3 9ER.

Glasgow: Gynaecological Clinic, Glasgow Royal Infirmary, Rottenrow, Glasgow, G4 0NA.

   also: Western Infirmary and Stobhill General Hospital.

   also: Royal Maternity Redlands Hospital, Great Western Road.

Leeds: MRC Mineral Metabolism Unit, General Infirmary.

Liverpool: Gynaecological Clinic, Women's Hospital, Catherine Street.

London: Menopause Clinic, Dept of Obstetrics and Gynaecology, Middlesex Hospital, Mortimer Street, W1.

also: The Menopause Clinic, Dept of Obstetrics and Gynaecology, King's College Hospital, Denmark Hill, SE5.

also: The Menopause Clinic, Dulwich Hospital, Dulwich, SE21.

also: The Menopause Clinic, Dept of Obstetrics and Gynaecology, Chelsea Hospital for Women, Doverhouse Street, SW3.

also: Dept. of Gynaecology, St Thomas's Hospital, SE1 7EH.

also: Royal Free Hospital, Pond Street, NW3.

also: St Mary's Hospital for Women, Marylebone, NW1.

also: Soho Hospital for Women, Soho Square, W1.

Manchester: Wythenshawe Hospital, Manchester 22.

also: Manchester General Hospital, Crumpsall, Manchester, M8 6RB.

Nottingham: The Menopause Clinic, Dept of Obstetrics and Gynaecology, City Hospital, Hucknell Road.

Nuneaton: Dept of Obstetrics and Gynaecology, George Eliot Hospital, College Street.

Oxford: Dept of Obstetrics and Gynaecology, John Radcliffe Hospital.

Peterborough: Peterborough and District Hospital, Thorpe Road.

Sheffield: University Department, Jessop Hospital.

Stafford: Stafford General Infirmary, Dept of Obstetrics and Gynaecology.

Stockport: Department of Obstetrics and Gynaecology, Stepping Hill Hospital, Stockport.

Migraine

If you suffer from migraine you should consult your doctor but the Migraine Trust has been set up to research into the causes and cure of migraine and to give advice and assistance to sufferers.

Migraine Trust
23 Queen's Square
London WC1

You could also contact the

City Clinic
11 Bartholomew Close
London EC1

Probation service

Probation officers also give help and advice in cases of family dispute including divorce. You will find their addresses in the telephone book.

Social security benefits

Leaflets about benefits are available from local social security offices or the Post Office. This is not an easy area to understand and the social services departments should be able to help you decide what you are entitled to.

Voluntary bodies

Concerned with the education and training of women

Freelance Work for Women
91 Parkway
London NW1

Objects: To promote home-based and part-time professional work for those unable to work a conventional office day; it also aims to improve and maintain the standard of work and to obtain current market rates for work so done.

Society for Promoting the Training of Women
Court Farm
Hedgerley
Bucks.

This society makes interest-free loans to women students for tuition fees and/or maintenance expenses whilst taking a recognized training. Loans are repaid after completion of training by monthly instalments which are normally at the rate of 15 per cent of the trainee's salary. Loans must be personally guaranteed or, in some cases, the Committee accept an endowment policy instead of a personal guarantor. Applications are considered by the Society's Committee who meet in London, usually once a month. Applicants are interviewed at these meetings.

The Over Forty Association for Women Workers
Grosvenor Gardens House
Grosvenor Gardens
London, SE1 0BS

Object: To provide employment and housing for the benefit of women workers of small incomes, particularly older women.

Concerned to help marriages under strain

The National Marriage Guidance Council
Herbert Gray College
Little Church Street
Rugby

Objects: The NMGC is concerned primarily with marriage and family relationships, and believes that the well-being of society is dependent on the stability of marriage. Its objectives are:

. 1. To provide a confidential counselling service for people who have difficulties or anxieties in their marriages or in other personal relationships.

2. To provide an education service in personal relationships for young people, engaged and newly married couples and parents.

3. To equip men and women to do this work by means of a national system of selection, training, tutorial support and supervision.

4. To publish and distribute literature on a wide variety of topics relating to marriage and family life.

5. To provide courses and conferences for teachers, ministers of religion, youth leaders and others and to co-operate with workers in related fields.

Concerned with the one parent family or those who have problems claiming benefits

Mothers in Action
Munro House
9 Poland Street
London W1

Objects: To press for improvement in the status of and facilities for unsupported mothers and their children by representation to local authorities or government departments and by specially conducted campaigns.

To disseminate information of special interest to unsupported mothers, and similarly to encourage their personal contribution by current research into their problems.

Gingerbread – same address as Mothers in Action.

Child Poverty Action Group
1 Macklin Street
Drury Lane
London

The National Council for the Unmarried Mother
and Her Child

became One Parent Families in November 1973

255 Kentish Town Road
London NW5 2LX

Objects: It is a national, non-denominational organization drawing together the voluntary and statutory agencies concerned. It works for improved social services for unmarried mothers and their children, tries to influence public opinion, and keeps a close watch on legislation affecting unmarried parents and their children. It's welfare department acts as a consultative agency and provides specialized advice to persons by putting them in touch with an appropriate social worker in their area or by providing direct help where necessary.

Other Voluntary bodies

National Citizens' Advice Bureaux
National headquarters
26 Bedford Square
London WC1

Objects: To make available for the individual accurate information and skilled advice on many of the personal problems that arise in daily life; to explain legislation; to help the citizen to benefit from and to use wisely the services provided for him by the State.

Pre-Retirement Association
Greenfield House
69–73 Manor Road
Wallington
Surrey SM6 0DQ

Objects: The Association was set up to continue and expand the work of the Preparation for Retirement Committee. It has a Council of Representatives of the organizations concerned with the different problems of retirement and an Association Membership of those wishing financially to support this new work. It is a servicing body, a central clearing-house to which information can be sent as fresh experience is gained, and from which interested individuals, commercial and industrial firms, civic and educational authorities and voluntary bodies can obtain reliable advice and information on request. Its purpose is to encourage the realization of an opportunity through timely thought and action – recognizing that preparation for retirement must be a voluntary matter for each individual.

MIND (National Association for Mental Health)
22 Harley Street
London W1

Objects: MIND aims to promote good mental health through public and professional education. It is an active pressure group for better services for, and prevention of, mental illness and handicap.

For additional information and help:

The Health Education Council
78 New Oxford Street
London WC1A 1AH